The Hughston Clinic
Sports Medicine Field
Manual

D1160293

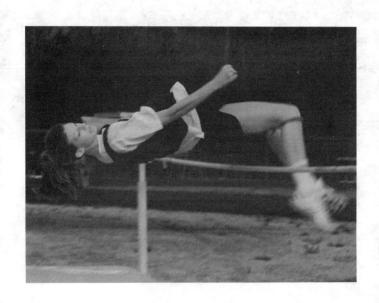

THE HUGHSTON CLINIC

Sports Medicine Field Manual

Champ L. Baker, Jr., M.D.
Editor-in-Chief

Fred Flandry, M.D.
Section Editor

John M. Henderson, D.O.
Section Editor

Hughston Sports Medicine Foundation, Inc.

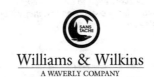

Williams & Wilkins
A WAVERLY COMPANY

BALTIMORE • PHILADELPHIA • LONDON • PARIS • BANGKOK
BUENOS AIRES • HONG KONG • MUNICH • SYDNEY • TOKYO • WROCLAW
1996

Editor: Darlene Cooke
Managing Editor: Sharon Zinner
Production Coordinator: Alethea H. Elkins
Book Project Editor: Robert D. Magee
Text Designer: Susan Blaker
Cover Designer: Karen Klinedinst
Typesetter: Maryland Composition
Printer: Courier
Binder: Courier

351 West Camden Street
Baltimore, Maryland 21201-2436 USA

Rose Tree Corporate Center
1400 North Providence Road
Building II, Suite 5025
Media, Pennsylvania 19063-2043 USA

RC1211
.H84
1995

Copyright © 1996 Williams & Wilkins

All rights reserved. This book is protected by copyright. No part of this book may be reproduced in any form or by any means, including photocopying, or utilized by any information storage and retrieval system without written permission from the copyright owner.

Accurate indications, adverse reactions, and dosage schedules for drugs are provided in this book, but it is possible that they may change. The reader is urged to review the package information data of the manufacturers of the medications mentioned.

Printed in the United States of America

Library of Congress Cataloging in Publication Data

The Hughston Clinic sports medicine field manual / Champ L. Baker,
   Jr., editor-in-chief : Fred Flandry, section editor ; John M.
   Henderson, section editor.
        p.   cm.
      Companion v. to: The Hughston Clinic sports medicine book / Champ
   L. Baker, editor-in-chief.   1995
      Includes index.
      ISBN 0-683-00310-0
      1. Sports medicine—Handbooks, manuals, etc.   I. Baker, Champ L.
   II. Flandry, Fred.   III. Henderson, John M. (John McKenzie), 1951—
      IV. Hughston Orthopaedic Clinic.
      [DNLM: 1. Sports Medicine—handbooks.   2. Athletic Injuries—
   handbooks.   QT 29 H894 1995]
   RC1211.H84   1995
   617.1′027—dc20
   DNLM/DLC
   for Library of Congress   95-25585
                                                                  CIP

The Publishers have made every effort to trace the copyright holders for borrowed material. If they have inadvertently overlooked any, they will be pleased to make the necessary arrangements at the first opportunity.

96 97 98 99
1 2 3 4 5 6 7 8 9 10

Reprints of chapters may be purchased from Williams & Wilkins in quantities of 100 or more. Call Isabella Wise in the Special Sales Department, (800) 358-3583.

This is dedicated to athletes everywhere,
the source of our inspiration and education.

DBCW - AEY 4549

JUN 12 1996

v

PREFACE

The true sports medicine professional practices his or her art on the sidelines of the playing field and in the locker room, not in the laboratory. Research is an integral part of the treatment of athletic injuries; however, in the field of sports medicine, the laboratory is on the field. This book, based on The Hughston Clinic's research and experience, was envisioned as a working guide for practitioners of sports medicine.

Sports medicine encompasses the total care of the athlete. This handbook is intended to assist you, the sports medicine professional who is actively engaged in the treatment of athletic injuries and diseases. You are provided with basic information in a condensed form to help you evaluate an injury or illness and develop a treatment plan for most of the problems an athlete will encounter. It will allow you to discuss with athletes and their parents the diagnosis, prognosis, and reasoning behind the treatment plan you have devised to promote a safe return to sport activity in the shortest possible time.

The reader can supplement this handbook with *The Hughston Clinic Sports Medicine Book*, which covers the same topics in greater detail, along with many other topics of interest to those who care for the athlete.

C. L. B.
Columbus, Georgia
1995

ACKNOWLEDGMENTS

I acknowledge the contributions of the residents, fellows, and staff at the Hughston Clinic, whose previous work was condensed into this handbook. I also thank Dr. Jack Hughston, whose lifelong involvement in sports and sports medicine has inspired us all.

In the actual production of this book, I wish to acknowledge the fine work of Dan Faber, who helped condense *The Hughston Clinic Sports Medicine Book* to this smaller, concise handbook form. The result of his writing skills were superbly consolidated and edited by Leslie Neistadt, who helped define the scope of the project and make it meaningful.

Major acknowledgment goes to Darlene Cooke of Williams & Wilkins, who had the vision for this handbook many months ago when *The Hughston Clinic Sports Medicine Book* was first being discussed. The idea of a smaller, "on-the-field" volume has been hers from the beginning, and we are pleased to be able to bring it to fruition. Sharon Zinner, also of Williams & Wilkins, ably directed the production process.

Special credit goes to Carol Capers, Judy Barr, and Yvonne Ehrhart whose illustrations and photographs can be found in this text as well as in the original book.

C. L. B.

CONTRIBUTORS

James R. Andrews, M.D.
Clinical Professor of Orthopaedics and Sports Medicine, University of Virginia Medical School, Charlottesville, Virginia
Clinical Professor, Department of Orthopaedic Surgery, University of Kentucky Medical Center, Lexington, Kentucky
Orthopaedic Surgeon, Alabama Sports Medicine and Orthopaedic Center, Birmingham, Alabama

Richard L. Angelo, M.D.
Assistant Clinical Professor of Orthopaedics, Team Physician, UW Huskies, University of Washington
Washington Orthopaedics and Sports Medicine, Kirkland, Washington

Michael J. Axe, M.D.
Co-Director, All Sports Clinic of Delaware, Newark, Delaware

Champ L. Baker, Jr., M.D.
The Hughston Clinic, P.C., Columbus, Georgia
Clinical Assistant Professor of Orthopaedics, Tulane University School of Medicine, New Orleans, Louisiana

Karl Lee Barkley II, M.D.
Family Practice, University Family Physicians, Charlotte, North Carolina
Team Physician, Davidson College, Davidson, North Carolina

Gene R. Barrett, M.D.
Mississippi Sports Medicine and Orthopaedic Center, Jackson, Mississippi

Major Kenneth B. Batts, D.O.
Director, Primary Care Sports Medicine, Family Practice Department, Tripler Army Medical Center, Honolulu, Hawaii

Paul W. Baumert, Jr., M.D.
Primary Care Sports Medicine, Kaiser Permanente, Overland Park, Kansas

Thomas N. Bernard, Jr., M.D.
Anderson, South Carolina

James L. Beskin, M.D.
Peachtree Orthopaedic Clinic, P.A., Atlanta, Georgia
Assistant Clinical Professor of Orthopaedics, Tulane University
School of Medicine, New Orleans, Louisiana

Kenneth M. Bielak, M.D.
Assistant Professor, Department of Family Medicine, Graduate
School of Medicine, University of Tennessee Medical Center at
Knoxville, Knoxville, Tennessee

Turner A. Blackburn, Jr., P.T., A.T.,C., M.Ed.
Cofounder and Director, Berkshire Institute of Orthopedic and Sports
Physical Therapy, Inc., Wyomissing, Pennsylvania
Adjunct Assistant Professor, Physical Therapy Program, University of
Miami School of Medicine, Miami, Florida

James R. Bocell, Jr., M.D.
Clinical Professor, Department of Orthopaedic Surgery, Baylor
College of Medicine, Houston, Texas

Thomas A. Boers, P.T., M.T.
Rehabilitation Services of Columbus, Columbus, Georgia

Mark R. Brinker, M.D.
Director of Orthopaedic Research, Department of Orthopaedic
Surgery, University of Texas Medical School at Houston,
Houston, Texas

Andrew A. Brooks, M.D.
Cedars-Sinai Medical Towers, Los Angeles, California

Douglas G. Browning, M.D., A.T.,C.
Assistant Professor in Family Medicine and Associate in Surgical
Sciences-Orthopedics/Sports Medicine, Bowman Gray School of
Medicine of Wake Forest University
Associate Team Physician, Wake Forest University, Winston-Salem,
North Carolina

Michael E. Brunet, M.D.
Professor of Orthopaedic Surgery, Tulane University School of
Medicine, New Orleans, Louisiana

Robert R. Burger, M.D.
Associate Director, Queen City Sports Medicine
Team Physician, Xavier University, The College of Mt. St. Joseph,
Wilmington College
Volunteer Clinical Instructor, Department of Orthopaedic Surgery,
University of Cincinnati, Cincinnati, Ohio

J. Kenneth Burkus, M.D.
The Hughston Clinic, P.C., Columbus, Georgia

Peter D. Candelora, M.D.
Consulting Staff, Shriners Hospital, Tampa, Florida
Chairman, Department of Surgery, Northbay Hospital, New Port
    Richey, Florida

William G. Carson, Jr., M.D.
Clinical Assistant Professor of Orthopaedic Surgery, University of
    South Florida College of Medicine, Tampa, Florida

Peter M. Cimino, M.D.
Omaha Orthopedic Clinic & Sports Medicine, P.C., Omaha, Nebraska

Massimo Cipolla, M.D.
Clinica Valle Giulia, Rome, Italy

Clark H. Cobb, M.D.
Faculty, Family Practice Residency Program, Co-Director, Primary
    Care Sports Medicine, Martin Army Hospital, Fort Benning,
    Georgia
Clinical Associate Professor of Family Practice, Uniformed Services
    University of the Health Sciences, Bethesda, Maryland

Mervyn J. Cross, MB., BS., M.D., F.R.A.C.S., F.A.Ortho A.
Crows Nest, New South Wales, Australia

Walton W. Curl, M.D.
Associate Professor of Orthopaedic Surgery, Bowman Gray School of
    Medicine of Wake Forest University
Director of Wake Forest University Sports Medicine Unit, Winston-
    Salem, North Carolina

Kenneth E. DeHaven, M.D.
Professor and Associate Chairman, Department of Orthopaedics,
    Director of Athletic Medicine, University of Rochester School of
    Medicine and Dentistry, Rochester, New York

R. Todd Dombroski, D.O.
Director of Primary Care Sports Medicine, Madigan Army Medical
    Center, Fort Lewis, Washington

Scott Dye, M.D.
Assistant Clinical Professor of Orthopaedic Surgery, University of
    California San Francisco, San Francisco, California

William Etchison, M.S.
Director of Industrial Relations and Wellness, Hughston Sports
    Medicine Foundation, Inc., Columbus, Georgia

Fred Flandry, M.D., F.A.C.S.
The Hughston Clinic, P.C.
Chairman, Department of Surgery, and Chief, Section of Orthopaedic
    Surgery, The Medical Center Hospital, Columbus, Georgia
Clinical Associate Professor, Department of Orthopaedic Surgery,
    Tulane University School of Medicine, New Orleans, Louisiana
Adjunct Assistant Professor in Small Animal Surgery and Medicine,
    College of Veterinary Medicine, Auburn University, Auburn,
    Alabama

Robert S. Franco, M.D.
First Coast Medical Group
Medical Director, Riverside Hospital Sports Medicine Program
Chairman, Riverside Orthopaedic Foundation, Jacksonville, Florida

Vittorio Franco, M.D.
Clinica Valle Giulia, Rome, Italy

Hugh A. Frederick, M.D.
Associate Attending Physician, Orthopaedic Surgery, Baylor
    University Medical Center, Dallas, Texas

Gerard T. Gabel, M.D.
Assistant Professor, Department of Orthopaedic Surgery, Baylor
    College of Medicine, Houston, Texas

Angelo Galante, M.D.
Staff Physician, Athleticare and Health Care Plan
Team Physician, Buffalo Blizzard, Buffalo Stampede, and Canisius
    College Ice Hockey, Buffalo, New York

Sandra Gibney, M.D.
Family Practice Resident, Medical Center of Delaware, Newark,
    Delaware

Joe Gieck, Ed.D., A.T.,C., P.T.
Head Athletic Trainer, Professor, Curry School of Education
Associate Professor, Orthopaedics/Rehabilitation, University of
    Virginia, Charlottesville, Virginia

John M. Graham, Jr., M.D.
Orthopaedic Surgeon, Charleston Orthopaedics, P.A.
Team Physician, College of Charleston
Clinical Instructor, Medical University of South Carolina, Charleston,
    South Carolina

Brian Halpern, M.D.
Medical Director/Chairman of the Board, Sports Medicine, New
    Jersey

Assistant Attending Physician, Sports Medicine Department, Hospital for Special Surgery

Assistant Attending Physician, New York Hospital, Cornell Medical Center, New York, New York

Clinical Assistant Professor, Sports Medicine, Robert Wood Johnson Medical School, University of Medicine and Dentistry of New Jersey, New Brunswick, New Jersey

James R. Harris, M.D.
Azalea Orthopedic and Sports Medicine Clinic, Tyler, Texas

David Harsha, M.D.
The Sports Medicine Institute of Indiana, Indiana Surgery Center, Indianapolis, Indiana

Jon M. Hay, M.Ed., A.T., C.
Head Athletic Trainer, Georgia Southwestern College, Americus, Georgia

John M. Henderson, D.O.
Director, Primary Care Sports Medicine, The Hughston Clinic, P.C., Columbus, Georgia

Jack H. Henry, M.D.
Clinical Professor of Orthopaedic Surgery, Columbia Presbyterian Medical Center, New York, New York

David L. Higgins, M.D.
Assistant Clinical Professor, Georgetown University School of Medicine, Washington, D.C.

Assistant Professor, Uniformed Services University of the Health Sciences, Bethesda, Maryland

Anne Hollister, M.D.
Adult Neuro Trauma Division, Rancho Los Amigos Medical Center, Downey, California

Kenny Howard, A.T.,C.
The Hughston Clinic, P.C., Auburn, Alabama

Tanya L. Hrabal, M.D.
Emergency Room Physician, Jacksonville, Florida

Jack C. Hughston, M.D.
Chairman of the Board, The Hughston Clinic, P.C., Columbus, Georgia

Professor Emeritus, Tulane University School of Medicine, New Orleans, Louisiana

Stephen C. Hunter, M.D.
The Hughston Clinic, P.C., Columbus, Georgia

Mary Lloyd Ireland, M.D.
Assistant Professor, College of Medicine (Orthopaedics), Department
   of Family Practice, Orthopaedic Consultant to Sports Teams,
   University of Kentucky
Director, Kentucky Sports Medicine Clinic, Lexington, Kentucky
Orthopaedic Consultant to Sports Teams, Eastern Kentucky
   University, Richmond, Kentucky

Joseph G. Jacko, M.D.
Southwest Orthopedic Institute, Dallas, Texas

Kurt E. Jacobson, M.D., F.A.C.S.
The Hughston Clinic, P.C., Columbus, Georgia

William D. Jones, P.T., C.S.C.S.
Human Performance and Rehabilitation Center, Columbus, Georgia

David M. Kahler, M.D.
Assistant Professor, Department of Orthopaedic Surgery, University
   of Virginia, Charlottesville, Virginia

Lee A. Kelley, M.D.
Peachtree Orthopaedic Clinic, P.A., Atlanta, Georgia

Gary Keogh, M.D., M.R.C.G.P., D.A., M.L.C.O.M., M.R.O.
Pennington, New Jersey

David B. Keyes, M.D.
Clinical Assistant Professor of Orthopaedic Surgery, University of
   Miami
Active Staff, Baptist Hospital of Miami
Courtesy Staff, South Miami Hospital, Miami, Florida

Bernard G. Kirol, M.D.
Nalle Clinic, Charlotte, North Carolina

Daniel R. Kraeger, D.O., A.T.,C.
Medical Director, Southern Wisconsin Sports Medicine Center
Medical Director, Mercy Sports Medicine Center, Janesville,
   Wisconsin

Robert E. Leach, M.D.
Professor of Orthopaedic Surgery, Boston University Medical School
Editor, American Journal of Sports Medicine, Boston, Massachusetts

Mark J. Leski, M.D.
Associate Professor of Family Practice, Director of Sports Medicine,
   Department of Family and Preventative Medicine, University of
   South Carolina, Columbia, South Carolina

Steven D. Levin, M.D.
Midwest Sports Medicine and Orthopaedic Surgery, Elk Grove
Village, Illinois

Stephen H. Liu, M.D.
Assistant Professor, Department of Orthopaedic Surgery, University
of California Los Angeles School of Medicine
Team Physician, UCLA Athletics, Los Angeles, California

Rene K. Marti, M.D.
Professor and Chairman, Orthopaedic Department, University of
Amsterdam, Amsterdam, Netherlands
Chief Consultant, Klinik Gut, St. Moritz, Switzerland

David F. Martin, M.D.
Assistant Professor of Orthopaedic Surgery, Bowman Gray School of
Medicine of Wake Forest University
Wake Forest University Sports Medicine Unit
Team Physician, Guilford College, Winston-Salem, North Carolina

Joseph A. Martino, M.D.
Cumming, Georgia

George M. McCluskey, Jr., L.A.T., PT
Rehabilitation Services of Columbus, Inc., Columbus, Georgia

George M. McCluskey III, M.D.
The Hughston Clinic, P.C., Columbus, Georgia
Clinical Assistant Professor, Department of Orthopaedic Surgery,
Tulane University School of Medicine, New Orleans, Louisiana

Leland C. McCluskey, M.D.
The Hughston Clinic, P.C., Columbus, Georgia

Frank C. McCue III, M.D.
Alfred R. Shands Professor of Orthopaedic Surgery and Plastic
Surgery of the Hand
Director, Division of Sports Medicine and Hand Surgery
Team Physician, Department of Athletics, University of Virginia,
Charlottesville, Virginia

Craig C. McKirgan, D.O.
Orthopaedic Surgeon, Center for Orthopaedics and Sports Medicine
Team Orthopaedic Surgeon, Indiana University of Pennsylvania,
Indiana, Pennsylvania

Thomas K. Miller, M.D.
Clinical Assistant Professor of Orthopaedic Surgery, University of
Virginia, Roanoke Program
Roanoke Orthopaedic Center, Roanoke, Virginia

Michael A. Oberlander, M.D.
Coastal Orthopaedic and Sports Specialists
Director, Sports Medicine, Health and Fitness Institute, Concord,
    California

Dianne Bazor Olszak, P.T.
Birmingham, Alabama

Arnold R. Penix, M.D.
Cincinnati, Ohio

William W. Peterson, M.D.
Memorial Clinic, Olympia, Washington

Robert M. Poole, M.Ed., P.T., A.T.,C.
Director, Human Performance and Rehabilitation Center, Inc.,
    Atlanta, Georgia
Clinical Professor of Physical Therapy, North Georgia College,
    Dahlonega, Georgia

Julie A. Pryde, M.S., P.T., A.T.,C.
Coordinator, Health and Fitness Institute, Center for Sports Medicine
Instructor, Department of Physical Therapy, Samuel Merritt College
Consultant, Intercollegiate Athletics, Saint Mary's College of
    California, Walnut Creek, California

Giancarlo Puddu, M.D.
Professor of Orthopaedics, University of Roma ''La Sapienza,''
    Rome, Italy

Reynold L. Rimoldi, M.D.
Las Vegas, Nevada

Lawrence D. Rink, M.D., F.A.C.C.
Clinical Professor of Medicine, Indiana University School of
    Medicine, Bloomington, Indiana

Lucien M. Rouse, Jr., M.D.
Assistant Professor, Department of Orthopaedics, Section of Athletic
    Medicine, University of Rochester School of Medicine and
    Dentistry, Rochester, New York

Carlton G. Savory, M.D.
The Hughston Clinic, P.C., Columbus, Georgia

Todd A. Schmidt, M.D., F.A.C.S.
The Hughston Clinic, P.C., Atlanta, Georgia

Alberto Selvanetti, M.D.
Clinica Valle Giulia, Rome, Italy

Robert M. Shalvoy, M.D.
Clinical Instructor in Orthopaedic Surgery, Brown University
Program in Medicine
Director, Ortho Sports New England, Providence, Rhode Island

Herbert L. Silver, P.T., E.C.S.
Physical Therapist, Human Performance and Rehabilitation Center,
Inc., Atlanta, Georgia
Clinical Faculty, Department of Physical Therapy, North Georgia
College, Dahlonega, Georgia

Patricia L. Skaggs, M.D.
The Hughston Clinic, P.C., Auburn, Alabama

Robert S. Skerker, M.D.
The Rehabilitation Institute, Morristown Memorial Hospital,
Morristown, New Jersey

Patrick A. Smith, M.D.
Team Physician, University of Missouri
Clinical Assistant Professor of Surgery, University of Missouri
School of Medicine, Columbia, Missouri

Robert O'Neil Snoddy, Jr., M.D.
Suwanee, Georgia

Tarek O. Souryal, M.D.
Director, Texas Sports Medicine Group, Dallas, Texas

Gregory W. Stewart, M.D.
Assistant Professor, Section of Physical Medicine and Rehabilitation,
Louisiana State University School of Medicine
Clinical Assistant Professor, Department of Orthopaedics, Tulane
University, New Orleans, Louisiana

Laura Stokes, M.S.
Columbus, Georgia

Timothy B. Sutherland, M.D.
Alabama Sports Medicine and Orthopaedic Center, Birmingham,
Alabama

William R. Sutton, M.D.
Wilmington, North Carolina

Suzanne Tanner, M.D.
Assistant Professor, Department of Orthopaedics and Pediatrics,
University of Colorado Health Services Center, Denver,
Colorado

Nancy J. Thompson, M.P.H., Ph.D.
Assistant Professor of Behavioral Science and Epidemiology, Rollins
School of Public Health, Emory University, Atlanta, Georgia

Paula R. Tisdale, O.T.R.
Staff Therapist, Sundance Rehabilitation Center, Columbus, Georgia

David Tremaine, M.D.
Director, Foot and Ankle Center at Anderson Clinic, Arlington,
Virginia
Clinical Assistant Professor of Surgery, Uniformed Services
University of the Health Sciences, Bethesda, Maryland

Hugh S. Tullos, M.D.
Baylor College of Medicine, Houston, Texas

John Turba, M.D.
President, Queen City Sports Medicine and Rehabilitation,
Cincinnati, Ohio

Tim L. Uhl, P.T.
Director of Physical Therapy, The Human Performance and
Rehabilitation Center, Columbus, Georgia
Adjunct Instructor of Clinical Physical Therapy, University of South
Alabama, Mobile, Alabama

John Uribe, M.D.
Associate Professor, Chief, Sports Medicine Division, Department of
Orthopaedics, University of Miami, Miami, Florida

Niek van Dijk, M.D.
University of Amsterdam, Amsterdam, Netherlands

J. William Van Manen, M.D.
Richmond, Virginia

Geoffrey Vaupel, M.D.
Medical Director, Institute for Sports Medicine, Davies Medical
Center, San Francisco, California

W. Michael Walsh, M.D.
Clinical Associate Professor of Orthopaedic Surgery, University of
Nebraska College of Medicine
Adjunct Graduate Associate Professor, School of Health, Physical
Education and Recreation, Team Orthopaedist for all sports,
University of Nebraska–Omaha, Omaha, Nebraska

Keith Webster, M.A., A.T.,C.
Director of Sports Relations, Hughston Sports Medicine Foundation,
Inc., Columbus, Georgia

Steven H. Weeden, B.A.
Medical Student, University of Texas Medical School at Houston,
    Houston, Texas

Barry L. White, P.T., M.S., E.C.S., R.E.P.T.
Physical Therapist, Clinical Electrophysiologic Specialist,
    Rehabilitation Services of Columbus, Columbus, Georgia

Franklin D. Wilson, M.D.
The Sports Medicine Institute of Indiana
Community Hospitals of Indianapolis Inc.
Assistant Professor of Orthopaedics, Indiana University Medical
    Center, Indianapolis, Indiana
Neutral Team Physician, National Football League

CONTENTS

1

Coverage of Games and Events

Team physicians provide coverage at professional, collegiate, high school, and recreational levels, as well as at events for special athletes. The organized professional team physician often is contracted to attend team events and care for individual team players. At recreational sports events, a physician may be present as an interested spectator or a supportive parent. Events organizers for special athletes usually seek physicians to cover their events because of the participants' health risks.

THE SPORTS MEDICINE TEAM

1. The team physician under contract, along with other physicians, athletic trainers, and therapists
2. The athletic trainer leads the team on the field with support of physicians and therapists, works under the direction and supervision of the team physician and acts to extend the physician's services

Comprehensive Injury Care Program

Working together, these professionals develop a comprehensive injury care program that includes the following:

1. Injury prevention strategies to reduce potential liability (eg, ensuring a safe playing area, teaching athletes proper conditioning exercises, taking appropriate precautions to prevent potentially fatal heat-related illnesses)
2. Proper, accurate assessment of injury type and severity
3. Appropriate first aid, including emergency plan and injury treatment
4. Determining if and when an injured athlete can return to play
5. Referral of injured athlete, when indicated, to appropriate medical professionals via network of medical specialists and allied health professionals
6. Effective rehabilitation programs to return athletes to sports as quickly as possible with minimal risk of reinjury
7. Educational and counseling programs (eg, seminars about health issues)

MEDICAL EQUIPMENT

The athletic trainer has primary responsibility for most medical equipment brought to the game. The trainer's kit includes supplies needed to repair equipment, treat minor injuries, and meet emergency needs (Table 1–1).

The team physician can inventory and suggest supplies for the trainer's kit, providing additional items needed to evaluate and treat potential emergencies during competition. These items can include diagnostic instruments and supplies for life support in emergencies.

If an ambulance is present at sporting event, the sports medicine team may not need to supply all emergency equipment. A well-trained and well-supplied ambulance crew on the sidelines greatly enhances the sports medicine team's capabilities.

Before game time, the sports medicine team identifies the location and accessibility of communications services (eg, cellular or line phones, radio, etc) so additional support can be enlisted as necessary.

GAME COVERAGE PROTOCOL

On the field, the athletic trainer is the principal member of the sports medicine team. Any injury or problem is assessed first by the trainer, who can handle many of them alone, and who calls on the physician for help as needed. Even when the physician cares for an injury on the field, he or she continues to work closely with the trainer to take advantage of their combined skills and provide optimum initial treatment to the injured athlete.

Most often, sports physicians assess and treat routine injuries on the field, with triage and stabilization the key factors. The decision to return an injured player to competition is based upon an assessment of the subsequent effect on the player and on the possibility of further injury to that player.

Serious injuries may require the physician's presence on the field to treat life- and limb-threatening problems, such as acute reactions to heat, head and spine injuries that present as neurologic emergencies, severe orthopedic injuries, and cardiac and pulmonary distress. While these situations are rare, the team physician needs to know the availability and capability of nearby hospital and emergency-room support.

HIGH-SCHOOL COVERAGE

A comprehensive sport medicine approach is necessary to any high-school athletic program and is in the best interest of the student athlete. Although high-school and recreational-level sporting organizations usually cannot afford a sophisticated sports medicine team, they can still

Table 1–1. Supplies That a Physician Should Have on Hand at Athletic Events

Tape supplies (variety of size and type of tape, prewrap, tape adherent, tape remover, etc.)
Scissors
Wound closures
Adhesive bandages (various sizes)
Gauze pads (sterile) and rolls
Elastic bandages (various sizes)
Gloves (sterile and nonsterile)
Slings
Crutches
Plastic bags for ice (make sure that ice is available)
Cryotherapy unit
Splints
Tongue depressors (sterile and nonsterile)
Bite stick
Hemostats
Penlight
Otoscope/ophthalmoscope
Suture kit including antiseptic cleanser (alcohol, Betadine, etc.), local anesthetic, syringes, and needles of various gauges. (Needles, syringes, and anesthetic must be kept in a secure place in the physician's kit.)
Thermometer
Scalpel handle and blades
Eye wash and saline for contact lens wearers
Pocket mirror
Dental kit
Antibiotic ointment and powder
Hydrogen peroxide
Cotton-tipped applicators (sterile)
Eye black
Cloth compression sleeves (compressionette, stockinette, etc.)
Bee sting kit, including epinephrine syringe
Paper bag (for hyperventilation)
Padding material (various sizes for protection of injuries incurred during practice or games)
Device to remove the facemask from a football helmet (e.g., bolt cutters, "trainer's angel," etc.)
Emergency information forms (one for each athlete)
An index card outlining an emergency plan with the following information: location of telephone, 911 service availability, availability of ambulance service, accessibility of the event site for the ambulance
Emergency equipment: mask and airway for CPR, stethoscope, blood pressure cuff
Emergency equipment (may be in conjunction with local ambulance service): spine board, stretcher, sand bags, rigid cervical collar, oxygen

This list is not intended to be all-inclusive. Add or delete items as they fit your particular needs. Items such as biomedical waste containers and disinfectant solutions used to prevent the spread of blood-borne pathogens should be included at your discretion. Quantities are determined by the number of athletes participating. Be sure to have other personnel available who are qualified to use emergency equipment. Review procedures about handling the football player who sustains a head or neck injury.

be effectively covered by a physician volunteer who works closely with an athletic trainer.

Every high school should have a carefully planned program to provide optimal care for its injured student athletes. The ideal program comprises a full-time athletic trainer as on-site director, supported by a qualified team physician, both of whom work closely with the coaching staff and receive full support from school administration and parents.

KEY PEOPLE FOR HIGH-SCHOOL PROGRAMS

The key people involved in establishing, running, and evaluating a comprehensive sports medicine program include

1. School administrators, who must commit to providing the best possible health care for students who participate in competitive athletics and extracurricular activities
2. Parents and athletic booster club members, who are often the driving force behind establishing a sport medicine program at their school and also a great resource for fund-raising efforts to acquire necessary facilities, equipment, and supplies
3. A team physician (selected by the school administration) who provides medical care and supervises the program and who must be well informed about the special demands and current practice of sports medicine
4. A daily on-site program director whose presence on the "front lines" is key to making the program succeed, who answers to the school and works closely with the team physician, and who in most cases, is a full-time, nationally certified athletic trainer who fulfills state regulatory requirements.

RESPONSIBILITIES OF THE ON-SITE DIRECTOR

1. Developing policy and procedure guidelines with school administrators
2. Organizing preparticipation physical examinations
3. Coordinating practice and event coverage
4. Maintaining accurate injury and treatment records
5. Keeping the supervising physician updated as to the condition of injured athletes
6. Maintaining a supply inventory and operating within a budget
7. Updating and revising protocols with the physician

Preparticipation Evaluation of Athletes

FUNCTIONS OF THE PREPARTICIPATION SCREENING EXAMINATION

1. Meeting legal and insurance requirements related to athletic participation
2. Determining athlete's general health
3. Evaluating athlete's level of physical conditioning
4. Assessing potential participant's physical maturity
5. Detecting conditions that may limit or contraindicate participation
6. Detecting conditions that may predispose to injury and allowing for rehabilitation of these injuries
7. Serving as baseline for determining when injured athlete may return to play
8. Affording opportunity for health education

LEGAL REQUIREMENTS

Legal requirements for the examination vary from state to state and with the level of athletic competition

1. Frequency often specified, most commonly once a year
2. Specific form may be available or standard form may need to be created
3. Criteria for exclusion from participation may be delineated
4. Athlete's parents may need to authorize emergency medical treatment
5. Health care providers who can perform examination may be specified
6. Minor must have parental permission for examination

Findings and recommendations for participation should be carefully documented. However, the physician's recommendations on participation are not the final authority. Ultimately, that decision rests with the athlete or the athlete's parents.

EXAMINATION PROTOCOL

1. Ideally, schedule examination several weeks before season begins to allow for correction or rehabilitation of any detected condition

2. May perform examination within individual or office-based system or group or station system
3. Office-based examination:
   a. Advantages: more privacy, easier accessibility of medical records, closer examiner-athlete relationship, and more comprehensive health care for athlete, in addition to meeting participation requirements
   b. Disadvantages: higher cost, more time required, and increased demand for providers
4. Group or station format:
   a. Extremely time efficient and may reduce costs significantly
   b. Allows coaches, trainers, and other athletic personnel to be involved
   c. Impersonal and requires much coordination

MEDICAL HISTORY

The most important part of the examination is the medical history (Table 2-1), an information-gathering process that should include the athlete's parents. The athlete is asked about the following:
1. General health, medical illnesses, medications, allergies, immunizations, surgical history, and details of any hospitalizations
2. Personal and family history of any cardiovascular disorders (eg, exertional syncope, chest pain, shortness of breath)
3. Previous musculoskeletal injuries and their present status
4. History of neurologic injuries (particularly any injuries resulting in concussion)
5. Previous heat or cold injuries
6. Menstrual history and possibility of pregnancy for female athletes

PHYSICAL EXAMINATION

1. Measure height, weight, resting pulse, pulse rate after exercise if time permits, and blood pressure; assess visual and dental status
2. Inspect skin and examine head, eyes, ears, nose, throat, heart, lungs, abdomen, and genitalia
3. Assess musculoskeletal system for ROM of major joints, gross instability, and flexibility; may also include specialized tests of flexibility, strength, power, speed, endurance, and body composition

LABORATORY SCREENING

Laboratory screening (urinalysis, hemoglobin measurement, or tuberculin tine test) is not recommended by the American Academy of Pediatrics

Table 2–1. History Questions for Athletic Physicals

Illness

Are you currently seeing a doctor for a medical problem?

Have you ever had:

Asthma or shortness of breath?

Allergies?

Bronchitis?

Epilepsy?

Hepatitis?

Mononucleosis?

Diabetes?

Heat illness or cramps?

Anemia?

Hernia?

High or low blood pressure?

Ulcer?

Tendency to bleed excessively?

Sickle cell disease or trait? [blacks only]

Do you tire easily?

Have you ever had chest pains or difficulty breathing, or passed out while exercising?

Do you have frequent or repeated backaches or strains?

Do you have frequent or repeated headaches?

Have you ever been told that you have a heart murmur, an irregular heartbeat, or any heart disease?

Have you ever been knocked out (unconscious)?

Have any members of your family had a ''heart attack,'' ''heart problems,'' or died before age 50?

Do you wear glasses or contact lenses?

Are you blind or partially blind in either eye?

Do you have any hearing problems?

Do you have any dentures or partials?

Do you smoke cigarettes or chew tobacco?

Males: Have you ever had a hydrocele?

　　　　Are you missing a testicle?

Females: Are you pregnant?

　　　　Do you have any menstrual disorders?

Medications

Are you taking any medications?

Are you allergic to any medications?

Injuries

Have you ever had a concussion, seizure, or convulsions?

Have you ever injured your: Neck?

　　　　　　　　　　　　　Nose?

　　　　　　　　　　　　　Throat?

　　　　　　　　　　　　　Eyes or ears?

　　　　　　　　　　　　　Head, arms or shoulders?

　　　　　　　　　　　　　Knees, ankles or legs?

　　　　　　　　　　　　　Chest or back?

　　　　　　　　　　　　　Abdomen or stomach?

Operations

Have you *ever* had any surgery or operation?

Are you missing any organ (eye, kidney, lung, etc.)?

Please record any *yes* answers.

Table 2–2. Classification of Sports

Contact/Collision	Softball
Boxing	Squash, handball
Field hockey	Volleyball
Football	**Strenuous Noncontact**
Ice hockey	Aerobic dancing
Lacrosse	Crew
Martial arts	Fencing
Rodeo	Field events:
Soccer	Discus
Wrestling	Javelin
Limited Contact/Impact	Shot put
Baseball	Running
Basketball	Swimming
Bicycling	Tennis
Diving	Track
Field events:	Weightlifting
High jump	**Moderately Strenuous Noncontact**
Pole vault	Badminton
Gymnastics	Curling
Horseback riding	Table tennis
Skating (ice or roller)	**Nonstrenuous Noncontact**
Skiing:	Archery
Cross country	Golf
Downhill	Riflery
Water	

(American Academy of Pediatrics: Recommendations for participation in competitive sports. Reproduced by permission of Pediatrics. *81*:737, 1988.)

CLEARANCE FOR ACTIVITY

Clearance for activity is probably the most difficult, and the most important, decision the physician makes in the preparticipation evaluation. However, very few persons are actually disqualified from participation because of evaluation findings

To help determine whether athlete should be allowed to participate in particular sport, the American Academy of Pediatrics' Committee on Sports Medicine recommends, based on exercise intensity and injury potential of sport, the guidelines in Tables 2–2 and 2–3. Sports activities are classified as follows:

1. Contact/collision
2. Limited contact/impact
3. Noncontact (strenuous, moderately strenuous or nonstrenuous)

Final Disposition of the Examination

Limited to 1 of 3 recommendations:

1. Unrestricted clearance

2. Clearance with restrictions (following completion of evaluation or rehabilitation)
3. No clearance (ie, disqualification) from particular sport or classification

If additional evaluation or rehabilitation required, restrict athlete from participation until it is completed. If athlete requires medication for participation, note this fact and notify the on-site director to ensure that such medication is available.

When specific problem is found that may limit participation, consider several concerns:
1. Is athlete or any other participant at increased risk for injury?
2. If athlete can safely participate with treatment of problem, should limited participation be allowed during treatment?
3. If clearance denied for particular activity, are there any activities in which athlete could safely participate?
4. Finally, remember that recommendations based on the screening examination are just that: recommendations. Legal right to final decision on participation rests with athlete or with his or her parents.

DISQUALIFYING CONDITIONS

Atlantoaxial Instability

1. Athletes with documented atlantoaxial instability should not participate in any contact/collision or limited contact/impact sports or sports that place too much repetitive flexion or extension stress on cervical spine
2. If any neurologic signs or symptoms exist in athlete with atlantoaxial instability, strenuous activity is contraindicated

Acute Illness

1. Sports participation during acute illness assumes risks:
   a. Worsening illness or transmitting it to others
   b. Dehydration or other thermoregulatory problems
   c. More serious complications of infections, such as myocarditis
   Thus, limit athletic activity during febrile illness.
2. "Above the neck" symptoms (stuffy or runny nose, sneezing, scratchy throat): may proceed cautiously with activity
3. Fever or "below the neck" symptoms (myalgia, hacking cough, vomiting, diarrhea): no work out

Cardiovascular Abnormalities

1. Hypertension
   a. Although upper limit of normal BP in young athletes unknown, one criterion is:

Table 2–3. Recommendations for Participation in Competitive Sports

	Contact		Noncontact		
	Contact/Collision	Limited Contact/Impact	Strenuous	Moderately Strenuous	Nonstrenuous
Atlantoaxial instability	No	No	Yes*	Yes	Yes
Acute illness†					
Cardiovascular problems					
Carditis	No	No	No	No	No
Hypertension					
Mild	Yes	Yes	Yes	Yes	Yes
Moderate†					
Severe†					
Congenital heart disease‡					
Ocular disorders					
Absence or loss of function of one eye§					
Detached retina‖					
Inguinal hernia	Yes	Yes	Yes	Yes	Yes
Single kidney	No	Yes	Yes	Yes	Yes
Hepatomegaly	No	No	Yes	Yes	Yes
Musculoskeletal disorders†					
Neurologic problems					
History of serious head or spine trauma, repeated concussions, or craniotomy	†	†	Yes	Yes	Yes

Convulsive disorder					
Well-controlled	Yes	Yes	Yes	Yes	Yes
Poorly controlled	No	No	Yes¶	Yes	Yes**
Ovary					
Absence of one	Yes	Yes	Yes	Yes	Yes
Respiratory problems					
Pulmonary insufficiency	††	††	††	††	Yes
Asthma	Yes	Yes	Yes	Yes	Yes
Sickle cell trait	Yes	Yes	Yes	Yes	Yes
Boils, herpes, scabies	‡‡	‡‡	Yes	Yes	Yes
Splenomegaly	No	No	No	No	Yes
Absent or undescended testicle	Yes§§	Yes§§	Yes	Yes	Yes

* Swimming; no butterfly, breast stroke, or diving starts.

† Needs individual assessment.

‡ Patients with mild forms can be allowed a full range of physical activities; patients with moderate or severe forms, or who are postoperative, should be evaluated by a cardiologist before athletics participation.

§ Availability of eye guards approved by the American Society for Testing and Materials may allow competitor to participate in most sports, but this must be judged on an individual basis.

‖ Consult ophthalmologist.

¶ No swimming or weight lifting.

** No archery or riflery.

†† May be allowed to compete if oxygenation remains satisfactory during a graded stress test.

‡‡ No gymnastics with mats, martial arts, wrestling, or contact sports until not contagious.

§§ Certain sports may require protective cup.

(Reproduced with permission of Pediatrics—Vol 81. pg 738. Copyright 1988.)

125/80 mm Hg for ages 10–12 yrs
135/85 mm Hg for ages 13–15 yrs
140/90 (ie, adult standards) for those older than 15 yrs.

b. Athletes with severe, uncontrolled hypertension (diastolic pressure > 115 mm Hg) or target organ involvement: no participation in competitive sports
c. Controlled hypertension and no target organ disease: may compete in sports that make moderate to high dynamic and low static demands
d. Controlled hypertension but left ventricular hypertrophy or renal function impairment: may participate in low-intensity activities (bowling, golf)

2. Murmurs
   a. Benign, functional cardiac murmurs do not preclude sports participation
   b. Various maneuvers (deep inspiration, Valsalva's, and squat-to-stand) can differentiate benign from pathologic murmurs
   c. Mitral valve prolapse need not restrict athlete from participation unless accompanied by any of the following:
      (1) Moderate to severe mitral regurgitation
      (2) Family history of sudden death associated with mitral valve prolapse
      (3) History of syncope, chest pain, or arrhythmias exacerbated by exercise
   d. Evaluate further any questionable murmur and defer clearance

3. Hypertrophic cardiomyopathy
   a. Most common cause of sudden death in young athletes
   b. Persons with hypertrophic cardiomyopathy should not participate in competitive sports if they have any of the following:
      (1) Marked left ventricular hypertrophy or significant left ventricular outflow obstruction
      (2) Arrhythmias
      (3) History of syncope
      (4) History of sudden death in relatives with hypertrophic cardiomyopathy

4. Other
   a. Clearance guidelines for athletes with arrhythmias or other abnormalities in *16th Bethesda Conference on Cardiovascular Abnormalities in the Athlete*
   b. If questions about cardiovascular status remain after complete evaluation, refer to cardiologist

Vision Impairment

1. Athlete with best corrected visual acuity in 1 eye < 20/50 considered functionally one-eyed and prohibited from sports in which no eye protection can be effectively worn

2. In other sports with high risk of eye injury (eg, football, baseball, racquetball), one-eyed athletes may participate if they wear approved lensed eye guard
3. However, ultimate decision for participation made on individual basis after potential risks and longterm serious consequences discussed with all involved parties

Inguinal Hernia

1. Athlete with asymptomatic inguinal hernia need not be excluded from any activity
2. Symptomatic hernias may be affected by activity and are evaluated individually

Kidney Abnormalities

1. Athlete with abnormal solitary kidney should not participate in contact or collision sports
2. Athlete with normal solitary kidney may participate, but should be advised of potential risks and longterm consequences of losing solitary functioning kidney: dialysis, transplantation

Hepatomegaly and Splenomegaly

1. Enlarged liver or spleen that has surpassed bony protection of rib cage at risk for injury in contact or collision sports; restrict participation
2. Restrict athlete with splenomegaly from strenuous noncontact sports; splenic rupture has occurred after even mild trauma

Musculoskeletal Disorders

1. Examine athlete with history of musculoskeletal problems for swelling or other inflammation, ROM, and strength compared with uninjured side, and functional testing of injured area
2. Fracture: consider location, type, and risk of further damage in determining clearance; playing cast or splint to protect fracture may be feasible; if uncertainty remains, seek orthopedic consultation

Neurologic Disorders

1. Concussion
   a. Most common head injury: cerebral concussion
   b. No universally accepted guidelines yet established, but Colorado Medical Society Sports Medicine Committee has developed basic criteria for management of concussion in sports, which can help determine athlete's clearance status
2. Neurapraxia
   a. History of burner or stinger (nerve root or brachial plexus neurapraxia) need not limit participation if athlete completely asymptomatic and physical examination normal

b. Evaluate further history of recurrent neurapraxia in single season or cervical spinal cord neurapraxia with transient quadriplegia
3. Seizures
a. Allow athlete with well-controlled seizures unrestricted clearance, provided participation itself does not trigger seizure
b. Athletes with poorly controlled seizures should not participate in contact or other potentially dangerous sports until seizure free for at least 1 month and medications and neurologic findings stable

Gynecologic Disorders

1. May clear female competitors with evidence of eating disorder, amenorrhea, or osteoporosis for participation after further evaluation
2. Having only 1 ovary not a restriction from participation

Pulmonary Disorders

1. Asthma not a contraindication if appropriate medical treatment provided and symptoms controlled
2. More significant pulmonary insufficiency may limit activity

Sickle Cell Trait and Disease

1. Need not restrict athletes with sickle cell trait in activity
2. Those with sickle cell disease and significant anemia usually limited in exercise capacity

Dermatologic Disorders

Infectious dermatologic conditions (boils, herpes, impetigo, scabies) preclude participation in contact sports until no longer contagious

Testicular Abnormalities

1. Discourage male athletes with single functioning testicle from participating in contact or collision sports
2. May participate if risks clearly understood and approved protective cup used
3. Refer athlete with undescended testicle for further evaluation

Human Immunodeficiency Virus (HIV)

1. Although risk of HIV transmission in sport believed to be very low, no currently available research directly assesses risk
2. As more data become available, specific recommendations about HIV and sports participation can be made

PRIMARY OBJECTIVES OF THE FITNESS ASSESSMENT

1. To minimize sports attrition due to injury
2. To improve athletic performance
3. To identify weaknesses that may hinder athletic performance

SECONDARY OBJECTIVES OF THE FITNESS ASSESSMENT

1. To assess achievement of individual goals
2. To help motivate athletes
3. To provide opportunity for wellness counseling
4. To evaluate success of preseason conditioning program
5. To provide sport-specific athletic profiles that match athletes to sport
6. To explain relationship between sport's demands and musculoskeletal adaptations

GENERAL PROTOCOL

1. Perform fitness assessment annually in station-screening format at time of physical examination, at least 6 weeks before season starts
2. Tests and methods should be simple to perform, easy to measure, reproducible, and inexpensive
3. Testing methods should closely resemble movements and activities actually used in competition

RELEVANT ANTHROPOMETRIC CHARACTERISTICS

1. Compare height and weight with standard growth charts to identify growth abnormalities
2. Body composition (general health indicator) can be important in determining success in certain sports; skin fold measurements (easy, reproducible, inexpensive, accurate) perhaps best overall method for calculating body composition in preparticipation fitness assessment

PERFORMANCE PARAMETERS FOR FUNCTIONAL OR ATHLETIC ABILITY

1. Muscle strength: maximum force generated
2. Muscle power: force and velocity generated
3. Muscle endurance: number of repetitions

Muscle strength, power, and endurance important in basic movements of running, jumping, lifting, and throwing; absolute tests of these factors involve displacement of known mass or use of identical loads for all athletes; relative tests involve displacement of one's own body weight or use of external loads in proportion to each athlete's maximum strength

4. Flexibility: ability to move joint through its normal ROM; easily measured with goniometer
5. Speed: ability to move body mass over time; closely related to strength and power
6. Aerobic endurance: ability to exercise large muscle groups in rhythmic fashion over prolonged period of time

Table 2–4. Most Important Components of Performance in Various Sports

Event or Position	Absolute Strength	Relative Strength	Absolute Power	Relative Power	Aerobic Endurance	Anaerobic-Aerobic Endurance	Muscle Endurance
Football							
Offensive back	X		X	X		X	
Defensive back	X		X	X		X	
Interior lineman	X		X	X		X	
Wide receiver				X		X	
Tight end	X		X	X		X	
Line backer	X		X	X		X	
Quarterback				X		X	
Baseball			X	X		X	X
Basketball				X	X	X	
Soccer				X	X	X	
Field hockey		X	X	X	X	X	
Wrestling	X		X	X		X	X
Fencing				X			X

Track: Running Events			
100 m			X
200 m			X
400 m			X
800 m			X
1 mile (1,500 m)		X	
2 miles		X	
5,000 m		X	
10,000 m		X	
Marathon		X	
Track: Field events			
Shot put	X		
Discus	X		
Hammer throw	X		
Pole vault		X	
High jump		X	
Long jump		X	

(Berger, R. A.: Applied Exercise Physiology. Philadelphia, Lea & Febiger, 1982, pp. 238–268.)

7. Anaerobic endurance: ability to move large muscle groups for at least 1 min, but generally not more than 2 min
8. Agility: combined speed, power, and flexibility, and ability to rapidly change direction
9. Balance: body's coordinated neuromuscular response to maintain defined position of equilibrium in response to changing visual, tactile, or kinesthetic stimuli
10. Reaction time: ability to respond to a stimulus

INTERPRETING RESULTS OF THE FITNESS ASSESSMENT

1. Assess team and individual performances relative to standard norms and peers
2. In interpreting results, view each athlete's strengths and weaknesses in terms of the demands of his or her sport (Table 2–4).
3. Give recommendations to correct areas of weakness or deficiency
4. Recognize, however, that adequate performance on fitness assessment does not imply skill and that skill does not ensure performance on athletic field

3

Environmental Medicine for the Athlete

HEAT-RELATED ILLNESSES

Exertional heat illnesses are common in athletes. Predisposing factors are listed in Table 3–1.

MINOR HEAT ILLNESSES

Minor heat illnesses include heat edema, heat tetany, heat syncope, miliaria rubra (prickly heat), and heat cramps (Table 3–2). Significant sunburn is also considered a common heat-related injury.

Common presenting symptoms
1. Headache
2. Vomiting
3. Dizziness
4. Goose flesh
5. Muscle cramps
6. Chilling
7. Fatigue
8. Apathy

Most athletes with heat-induced illness have at least some of these complaints, but some collapse without warning.

Physical findings
1. Hyperpyrexia
2. Flushing
3. Tachycardia
4. Tachypnea
5. Oliguria
6. Hyperreflexia
7. Mydriasis
8. Hypotension
9. Dehydration

More seriously affected individuals may experience
1. Altered mental status

Table 3–1. Predisposing Factors to Heat Illness

Endogenous	*Exogenous*
Age (extremes)	Increased temperature
Dehydration	Increased humidity
Obesity	No breeze
Exercise	No cloud cover
Hypokalemia	Inaccurate temperature information
Alcohol	
Mid-day overeating	
Heart disease	
Sweat gland problems	
Drugs*	
History of heat injury	
Sunburn	

* Drugs that either increase endogenous heat production (tricyclic antidepressants, amphetamines, LSD, PCP, cocaine, etc.) or those that impair heat dissipation (anticholinergics, antihistamines, diuretics, tricyclic antidepressants, β-blockers) are associated with increased risk.

Table 3–2. Characteristics of Minor Heat Illnesses

Heat edema:	Benign, self-limited swelling of the hands and feet, usually seen in the first few weeks of acclimatization and resolves with cooling, elevation of the affected part, and light compression when necessary. Diuretics should be avoided.
Heat tetany:	Carpopedal spasm (probably secondary to the normal hyperventilation seen with increased temperature)
Heat syncope:	Function of decreased vasomotor tone and venous pooling with exercise and elevated body temperature. Decreased hydration also contributes, but aggressive fluid replacement may not be required.
Miliaria rubra:	Maculopapular, erythematous rash on clothed parts of body when keratin plugs block sweat gland pores or when the glands themselves swell. Proper hygiene is usually sufficient treatment.
Heat cramps:	Cramps of heavily worked muscle groups (lower extremity and abdomen in particular) that appear to wander since the entire muscle is usually not affected. They are usually associated with a whole-body salt deficiency. Treatment often entails sodium replacement (0.1% oral saline solution or IV normal saline).

2. Seizures
3. Coma

HEAT EXHAUSTION AND HEAT STROKE

However, heat exhaustion and heat stroke can be difficult to distinguish initially, as signs and symptoms of multiple organ system dysfunction seen with the latter may not become evident for hours or days. Any indication of renal, neurologic or hepatic injury during first 24 hrs, though, should lead to presumptive diagnosis of heat stroke. In hot weather, collapse of previously healthy person during physical exertion reflects heat stroke unless another cause obvious. Remember that lower temperature does not preclude heat stroke.

Early Management

1. Initiate rapid cooling immediately, trying to cool to core temperature of 102° F within the first 30–60 min
2. Transport patient to medical facility as soon as possible
3. Administer oxygen, monitor temperature, and establish IV access en route
4. Overly aggressive administration of IV fluids may not be required and can lead to overshoot hyponatremia and pulmonary edema

Hospital Management

1. First priority: airway, breathing, circulation management
2. Rapid cooling (0.15° C/min) to 102° F (39° C) by
   (a) Immersion in iced or tap water
   (b) Dousing patient with water
   (c) Applying ice packs or
   (d) Spraying patient with cool mist after removing restrictive clothing
   Spray and fan method is quick and easy and our preferred option.
3. Take precautions to prevent overshoot hypothermia or unmonitored rebound hyperthermia after cooling accomplished

Table 3–3. Historical Differentiating Features of Heat Exhaustion and Heat Stroke

	Heat Exhaustion	Heat Stroke
Body Temperature	Less than 102° F	More than 104° F
Mental Status Changes	No	Yes
Sweating	Yes	Usually absent, but may be excessive

4. Obtain baseline laboratory tests, chest radiograph, EKG: thermoregulatory mechanisms function abnormally for at least several days

Possible Laboratory Abnormalities

1. Primary respiratory alkalosis from hyperventilation and ↑ body temperature
2. Subsequent metabolic acidosis from ↑ glycolysis and lactic acid accumulation
3. Hypo- or hyperglycemia
4. Hypokalemia in early stages
5. Hyperkalemia later
6. Sodium levels vary widely with hydration status and treatment fluids
7. ↓ phosphate, calcium, and magnesium levels
8. ↑ liver function tests and bilirubin levels
9. White cell count may ↑, but platelets may ↓
10. Hypoprothrombinemia and hypofibrinogenemia may lead to disseminated intravascular coagulation
11. Marked ↑ creatine phosphokinase level after prolonged endurance exercise
12. Significant ↑ transaminase level after 24–48 hrs
13. Concentrated urine with ketones, protein, and myoglobin

Possible Complications of Heat Stroke

1. CNS disturbances: confusion, lethargy, depression, irritability, delirium, seizures, cerebellar deficits, and coma
2. Transient conduction disturbances on EKG
3. Low cardiac output, sinus tachycardia, heart block, and tachyarrhythmia, especially in cool-down period
4. ↑ pulmonary vascular resistance, pulmonary edema, adult respiratory distress syndrome, disseminated intravascular coagulation, or aspiration pneumonia
5. Azotemia, either renal or prerenal
6. Acute renal failure in 25% of exertional heat stroke patients
7. Hepatic disorders
8. Gastrointestinal dysfunction: nausea, vomiting, diarrhea, stress ulceration, or frank hemorrhage
9. Impaired hemostasis

Treatment of Complications

1. Early complications: prompt cooling and careful rehydration
2. Acute renal failure: fluids, furosemide, and mannitol
3. Lack of diuretic response, anuria, uremia or hyperkalemia: dialysis
4. Congestive heart failure: central monitoring and dopamine in extreme cases (avoid α agonists)

5. Dysrhythmias: establish Advanced Cardiac Life Support (ACLS) protocols
6. Combative patient: benzodiazepine sedation (avoid physical restraints)
7. Shivering or seizures: diazepam (Valium)
8. Antipyretics not effective in treating heat-related illnesses and can be detrimental to injured hepatic, renal, or gastrointestinal organs

Good Prognosis

1. Patient promptly evacuated and managed in appropriate medical facility
2. Body temperature rapidly reduced
3. Rehydration properly managed
4. Seizures and other complications controlled

Poorer Prognosis

1. Initial temperature >106° F
2. ↑ duration of hyperthermia
3. Coma >2 hrs or persisting after temperature has returned to normal
4. Oliguria, renal failure, hyperkalemia, and aspartate aminotransferase levels > 1000 IU

Postinjury Restrictions

Athletes with mild cases of heat stroke (no end-organ damage or dysfunction) should:
1. Avoid running, jumping, prolonged standing or walking, lifting >5 lbs, and any strenuous exertion
2. Limit exposure to adverse environmental conditions for 72 hrs
3. Avoid strenuous activity if body weight ↓ 5% or more while training
4. Ingest liberal amounts of fluids and food

Athletes suffering severe cases (end-organ damage or significant laboratory abnormalities) should:
1. Follow above restrictions for 72 hrs
2. Then exercise at their own pace and distance in wet bulb-globe temperatures below 86° F for the next 90 days (Table 3–4)
3. Be re-evaluated before resuming usual activities

PREVENTIVE MEASURES FOR HEAT ILLNESSES

1. Conditioning: endurance training
   a. ↑ sweat rate at given temperature
   b. ↓ core temperature at given levels of physical stress
   c. ↑ plasma volume
   d. ↓ heat storage

   Intense interval training, even in a cool environment, improves heat tolerance more than mild to moderate exercise if fluid balance maintained and factors that predispose to heat injury are avoided.

2. Acclimatization: 3–4 hrs/day exposure to work and heat for 10–14 days results in
   a. ↓ heart rate, rectal temperature, and perceived exertion
   b. ↑ plasma volume and sweat rate which
      (1) ↓ physiologic strain
      (2) ↑ ability to exercise in hot environment
      (3) ↓ incidence of some forms of heat illness
   However:
      (1) Even after becoming acclimatized, these adaptations lost in few days or wks of inactivity
      (2) Athletes arriving for competition on short notice are unacclimatized, regardless of physical condition
      (3) Acclimatization does not guarantee that athlete will be immune to heat illnesses

3. Fluid Replacement
   a. Training and acclimatization do not ↓ water needs
   b. Thirst: very poor indicator of hydration status
   c. "Mild dehydration" of 2–3% ↓ work capacity by 15–20%; losses of 4% may ↓ capacity by 30%
   d. For every L water lost
      (1) Rectal temperature ↑ by 0.3° C
      (2) Cardiac output ↓ by 1 L/min
      (3) Heart rate ↑ 8 BPM
   e. Drink before, during, and after exercising in heat to maintain fluid balance (cool to cold fluids absorbed best)
   f. If exercising >90 mins, need adequate replacement of water, carbohydrates, and electrolytes
   g. Intake recommendations:
      (1) 15–20 mins before exercising: 400–600ml (13–20oz) cold water or 4–8% carbohydrate-electrolyte beverage
      (2) During exercise: 200–300ml every 15–20 mins
      (3) After exercise: restore at least 80% of loss

4. Tools for Prevention
   a. Use wet bulb-globe temperature (Table 3–4) as guide in modifying activity
   b. Modify uniforms
   c. Change work-rest cycles
   d. Drink enough fluids
   e. Cooling spray
   f. Change practice time to avoid heat of day
   g. Educate athletes, coaches, supervisors, and parents about acclimatization, fluid replacement, proper clothing, and early recognition and treatment of suspected heat-related illnesses

Table 3–4. Wet Bulb–Globe Temperature (WBGT) and Recommended Activity Levels

WBGT		Activity
°C	°F	
15.6	60	No precautions
19–21	66–70	No precautions as long as water, salt, and food are easily available
22–24	71–75	Postpone sports practice, avoid hiking
24	76	Lighter practice and work with rest breaks
27	80	No hiking or sports
28	82	Only necessary heavy exertion with caution
30	85	Cancel all exertion for unacclimatized persons; avoid sun exposure even at rest
31.5	88	Limited brief activity for acclimatized, fit persons only

(Yarbrough, B. E., Hubbard, R. W.: Heat related illness. *In* Management of Wilderness and Environmental Emergencies. 2nd Ed. Edited by P. S. Auerbach and E. C. Geehr. St. Louis, C. V. Mosby, 1989.)

CHILDREN AND HEAT INJURY

Children may be at ↑ risk for heat-related injury because they
1. Gain heat more rapidly from environment
2. Sweat less effectively
3. Produce ↑ metabolic heat for given work load
4. Acclimatize more slowly than adults
5. Have ↑ mass to surface area ratio
6. Have ↓ renal tubular filtration rate
7. Often lack experience and judgment to perceive signs of impending heat injury

WOMEN AND HEAT INJURY

1. Thermoregulation may be compromised somewhat during prolonged exercise or heat exposure while in luteal phase of menstrual cycle
2. However, few differences exist between men and women in acclimatizing to heat

COLD INJURIES

Cold affects CNS, heart, lungs, and muscles. Shell—skin, muscles, and extremities—is affected first, resulting in ↓ circulation to guard and protect the body's core temperature. This can result in weak, stiff muscles, ↑ nerve conduction time, and ↓ athletic performance. Cold injuries render athletes more susceptible to second such injury.

PREDISPOSING FACTORS

1. Inadequate or wet clothing
2. Wind chill factor
3. Altitude
4. Moisture content of air
5. Injury
6. Alcohol consumption, age extremes, poor nutrition, fatigue, or medications
7. Use of tobacco or constricting garments

Hypothermia: core body temperature < 97° F (35° C)

Mild hypothermia: (core temperature between 90° F and 95° F [32° C and 35° C]) produces changes in mentation, best indicator of hypothermia

With severe hypothermia (core temperature < 90° F [32° C]), cardiovascular and CNS changes are the most serious consequences:

risk of ventricular fibrillation ↑
response to medical treatment ↓
↓ blood flow and ↑ blood viscosity impair mentation

Progressive Signs and Symptoms of Hypothermia

1. Complaints of cold and loss of interest in activity
2. Fine motor skills suffer, decision-making capabilities deteriorate, and the desire for sleep grows strong
3. Inability to be aroused
4. Physical examination: bradycardia, hypotension, muscle rigidity, and dilated pupils

Early Treatment

1. Mild hypothermia
   a. Move patient from cold environment to warmer one
   b. Remove all wet clothing after relocation
   c. Place external heat sources in areas of high heat loss (neck, armpits, groin)
   d. If external heat sources not available, have another person lie next to hypothermia victim
   e. Give oral hydration if patient alert
2. Severe hypothermia
   a. Rewarming patients in field controversial
   b. Evacuation to treatment facility mandatory
   c. Before initiating CPR, confirm absence of pulse for 1 min (may be difficult to detect pulse because of intense vasoconstriction, bradycardia, and shallow, irregular breaths)

Poor Outcome Factors

1. Body core temperature <82° F (28° C) or equal to ambient temperature
2. Submersion >50 min
3. Associated life-threatening injury
4. Elapsed time to definitive care >4 hrs

FROSTBITE

Frostbite, body's response to severe cold, occurs from direct freezing and from vascular changes that produce ischemia. Susceptible body parts: nose, ears, feet, fingers, and penis. At times, difficult to distinguish superficial from deep frostbite until thawing complete.

1. Superficial or first-degree frostbite
   a. White patches of frozen skin, but skin remains soft and resilient when depressed
   b. Wounds usually heal without permanent sequelae
2. Second-degree frostbite
   a. Bullous formation and edema within 24 hrs of rewarming
   b. Blisters dry within 7–10 days, leaving hard black eschar that separates in 3–4 wks, exposing delicate red skin
3. Third- and fourth-degree frostbite
   a. "Woody" frozen parts remain cool and mottled after rewarming
   b. Small, dark bullae form in few days or weeks (or sometimes not at all)
   c. Edema develops and resolves slowly
   d. Demarcation over 3–6 weeks, followed by mummification and spontaneous amputation of dead tissue

Treatment

1. Rewarm frostbitten areas only when no danger of refreezing
2. Sedate patient as needed and treat for metabolic acidosis, hypoxia, and hypotension
3. Keep patient in bed until edema subsides and blisters dry
4. Place lamb's wool between toes to prevent maceration
5. Delay sterile escharotomy until eschar starts to separate
6. Update tetanus immunization if necessary
7. Prohibit nicotine products
8. Administer antibiotics
9. Start gentle ROM as soon as possible

CHILBLAIN

Chilblain, or pernio, is caused by cool temperatures and high humidity. This neurocirculatory condition produces superficial lesions that heal quickly.

Signs and Symptoms

1. Dermatitis
2. Itching
3. Skin ulcerations
4. Chronic inflammation

Trench foot results from prolonged exposure (>12 hrs) of wet feet to temperatures between 32° F and 50° F (0° C and 10° C).

PREVENTION OF COLD INJURIES

1. Protect body from heat loss with
   a. Layered clothing (wool, wool-synthetic blends, polypropylene, or capeline)
   b. Outer jacket (GoreTex, nylon, or 60–40 cloth)
   c. Face mask, balaclava, or ski-type neck warmer
   d. Cap to cover head
   e. Ski goggles to protect eyes
   f. Polypropylene hand and foot coverings using GoreTex or nylon
2. ↑ heat production
3. Warm-up indoors when possible
4. Perform longer warm-ups during cold weather

HIGH-ALTITUDE ILLNESS

Terrestrial elevations of 1500–3500m (5001–11,480 ft) are considered high altitude. Elevations between 3500 and 5500m (11,480–18,000 ft) are very high altitude. Extreme altitudes are those higher than 5500m (18,000 ft).

Illnesses or syndromes associated with exposure to high terrestrial altitudes can be grouped according to severity:

1. Minor, rarely disabling, and nonfatal
   a. High-altitude systemic edema
   b. High-altitude retinal hemorrhages
   c. High-altitude flatus expulsion
   d. Ultraviolet keratitis
   e. Altitude throat
2. Disabling, but nonfatal
   a. Acute mountain sickness
   b. Chronic or subacute mountain sickness
   c. High-altitude deterioration

ACUTE MOUNTAIN SICKNESS

Acute mountain sickness, most common of all altitude illnesses, rarely occurs below 2440m (8000 ft), with most people not experiencing symptoms until 3050–3660m (10,000–12,000 ft).

Symptoms

1. Headache
2. Lassitude
3. Anorexia
4. Malaise
5. Weakness
6. Dyspnea on exertion
7. ↓ urine output
8. Facial warmth and flushing for the 1st 24–48 hrs
9. Tinnitus and vertigo
10. Difficulty sleeping, frequent periods of wakefulness, and strange dreams

Clinical Signs

1. Tachypnea
2. Tachycardia
3. Cheyne-Stokes respirations
4. Ataxia

Treatment

1. Mild to moderate cases (symptomatic relief)
   a. Rest
   b. Light diet
   c. Fluids
   d. Analgesics for headache
2. Severe cases
   a. Rapid descent to low altitude
   b. Supplemental oxygen, especially during sleep
   c. Pharmacologic therapy: dexamethasone (Decadron) 8mg initially, then 4mg q6 hrs

   Prevention: Slow acclimatization by 2- to 4-day sojourn at intermediate altitude (1830–2440m) and then gradual ascent to higher elevations

Possible Pharmacologic Prophylaxis

1. Acetazolamide (Diamox) 250mg q6–12 hrs (or 500mg/day of sustained-release formulation), beginning 1–2 days before ascent and continuing at high altitude for 2 or more days; mild diuretic, so maintain adequate hydration
2. Dexamethasone (Decadron) 4mg q6 hrs
3. Combined acetazolamide 250mg bid and dexamethasone 4mg qid more effective than either alone

HIGH-ALTITUDE CEREBRAL EDEMA

High-altitude cerebral edema, a life-threatening form of altitude illness, affects estimated 1% of high-altitude travelers and usually occurs at altitudes above 3660m (12,000 ft).

Clinical Presentation (progressive neurologic signs and symptoms)

1. Truncal ataxia, lassitude, and altered sensorium may progress to obtundity, stupor, and coma
2. Headache, nausea, vomiting
3. Paresthesias, diplopia, and vertigo
4. Focal neurologic deficits (eg, cranial nerve abnormalities, aphasia, hemiparesis) mimicking stroke
5. Retinal hemorrhages and papilledema on fundoscopic examination
6. Loss of consciousness may occur within 12 hrs, but usually takes 1–3 days

Treatment

1. Critical: early recognition and prevention of progression
2. Immediate, rapid descent once symptoms recognized
3. Dexamethasone, if available, 4–8mg IV, IM, or PO, followed by 4mg q6 hrs
4. Supplemental oxygen if available
5. Evacuation to hospital for aggressive management
   Prognosis: Favorable if above steps taken

HIGH-ALTITUDE PULMONARY EDEMA

High-altitude pulmonary edema, a severe, potentially life-threatening form of high-altitude illness, usually occurs within 1st 2–4 days of ascent to altitude higher than 2500m (8200 ft) and begins on 2nd night at altitude.

Early Warning Signs

1. ↓ exercise performance
2. Tachypnea, even at rest
3. Fatigue
4. Weakness
5. Headache, anorexia, and lassitude
6. Dry cough progressing to productive cough
7. Cyanosis
8. Audible congestion
9. Progressive deterioration: mental status changes, ataxia, and ↓ consciousness

Clinical Manifestations

1. Low-grade fever
2. Tachycardia and tachypnea in severe cases
3. Unilateral or bilateral rales
4. EKG changes consistent with acute pulmonary hypertension and

right-sided heart strain (ie, right axis deviation, right bundle branch block, cor pulmonale, or right ventricular hypertrophy)

5. ↑ mean pulmonary artery pressure and pulmonary vascular resistance with low to normal capillary wedge pressure
6. Chest radiographs consistent with noncardiogenic pulmonary edema
7. ABG analysis: severe hypoxia, hypocapnia, and acute respiratory alkalosis from hyperventilation

Treatment

1. Rapid descent to lower altitude
2. Supplemental oxygen at 6–12 L/min
3. Hospitalization for severely affected persons; manage as noncardiogenic pulmonary edema
4. Nifedipine 20mg q8 hrs for prophylaxis in susceptible persons and as emergency supplement

4

Head and Facial Injuries

PATHOPHYSIOLOGY OF HEAD INJURIES

The skull and brain are generally injured in 1 of 2 ways:
1. Coup injury: an object strikes the resting but movable head, causing maximal brain injury beneath point of impact
2. Contrecoup injury: the moving head strikes a nonmoving object, usually producing maximal brain injury on the side opposite impact

Brain injury results from rotational (angular) or translational (linear) forces.
1. Rotational forces → shearing stresses → loss of consciousness
2. Translational forces → compressive forces → skull fracture, intracranial hematoma, and cerebral contusion rather than unconsciousness
3. Brain tolerates compressive stress better than tensile or shearing stress
4. Degree of brain injury related to position and motion of head at time of impact

Classify head injuries as focal or diffuse.

FOCAL BRAIN INJURIES

Cerebral Contusion

1. Ill-defined area of small hemorrhages, necrosis, and edema
2. Occurs most often from acceleration-deceleration (translational) force (eg, when athlete's head strikes ground)
3. Results in typical contrecoup lesion: local loss of brain function and creation of mass effect compressing adjacent brain tissue

Intracerebral Hematoma

1. Occurs deep within brain
2. Often results from force applied to head over small area
3. Symptoms determined by size and location of hematoma
   a. Decreased level of consciousness
   b. Severe persistent headaches
   c. Amnesia

Epidural Hematoma

1. Results from tear of middle meningeal artery with temporal skull fracture
2. Most potentially life threatening of focal head injuries; high mortality and morbidity, even with early recognition and treatment
3. Death from mass effect of rapidly expanding hematoma, which causes brain herniation
4. Classic presentation
   a. Loss of consciousness at time of injury followed by lucid period of variable length
   b. Then rapid deterioration: severe headache and decreasing level of consciousness
   c. Coma and death may occur within 15–30 min
5. However, classic presentation in only 12–33% of patients, thus absence of same does not exclude diagnosis
6. Brain injury usually not significant, and complete neurologic recovery possible if hematoma recognized promptly and treated surgically

Subdural Hematoma

1. Occurs when bridging veins between brain and dura are torn or when injury results in laceration of brain parenchyma
2. Acute Presentation
   a. Brief or no lucidity
   b. Athlete rendered unconscious at time of injury generally remains unconscious
   c. Bleeding and associated swelling create enlarging mass that may cause nausea, vomiting, seizures, and hemiparesis
   d. Ipsilateral ocular ptosis or pupillary dilatation from herniation compressing brain stem and cranial nerves
3. Subacute Presentation
   a. Develops over 1 to 3 days from slow bleeding and less parenchymal injury
   b. Initial head injury often assumed insignificant
   c. Generalized headache and dizziness to confusion, memory loss, and personality changes
   d. Suspect if athlete not steadily improving
4. Treatment: rapid evacuation of hematoma best ↓ chance of serious complications and death
5. Prognosis
   a. Mortality rates as high as 70%
   b. Only 11% of patients return to work
   c. Possibility of returning to contact sports extremely small

Table 4–1. Grading Scale for Concussions

Grade	Symptoms
Grade I (mild)	Confusion
	No amnesia
	No loss of consciousness
Grade II (moderate)	Confusion
	Amnesia
	No loss of consciousness
Grade III (severe)	Loss of consciousness

(Adapted from Colorado Medical Society: Report of the Sports Medicine Committee: Guidelines for the management of concussion in sports (revised). Denver: Colorado Medical Society, 1991.)

DIFFUSE BRAIN INJURIES

Concussion

1. Most common head injury and sometimes most difficult to recognize
2. ''Traumatically induced alteration in mental status''
3. Hallmarks: confusion and amnesia in presence or absence of consciousness
4. Classification systems for grading severity based on duration of unconsciousness, duration of post-traumatic amnesia, or both (Table 4–1)
5. Suggested management guidelines for return to competition after concussion based on presence or absence of confusion, amnesia, and loss of consciousness. (Table 4–2)

Diffuse Axonal Injury

1. Diffuse axonal injuries represent more severe brain dysfunction
2. Prolonged traumatic coma occurs, with loss of consciousness for several hours
3. Residual neurologic, psychologic, or personality deficits often result

GENERAL PRINCIPLES OF ON-FIELD MANAGEMENT

1. Presume every unconscious athlete and any conscious athlete who complains of neck pain, numbness, weakness, or paralysis has cervical spine injury until proven otherwise; stabilize spine until radiographic evaluation done
2. Assess ABCs (airway, breathing, circulation)
3. Perform baseline neurologic evaluation

Table 4–2. Guidelines for Return to Play After Concussion

Grade	First Concussion	Second Concussion	Third Concussion
Grade I (mild)	May return to play when asymptomatic for at least 20 min	Terminate contest/practice; may return to play if asymptomatic for at least 1 week	Terminate season; may return to play in 3 months if asymptomatic
Grade II (moderate)	Terminate contest/practice; may return to play when asymptomatic for 1 week	Consider terminating season, but may return to play if asymptomatic for 1 month	Terminate season; may return to play next season if asymptomatic
Grade III (severe)	Terminate contest/practice and transport to hospital; may return to play 1 month after two consecutive asymptomatic weeks; conditioning allowed after 1 asymptomatic week	Terminate season	Regardless of grade a season is terminated by any abnormality on CT or MRI consistent with brain contusion or other intracranial lesion

(Adapted from Colorado Medical Society: Report of the Sports Medicine Committee: Guidelines for the management of concussion in sports (revised). Denver: Colorado Medical Society, 1991.)

    a. Use AVPU method (Glasgow coma scale) to determine level of consciousness: A, alert; V, responds to verbal stimulus; P, responds to painful stimulus; U, unconscious

    b. Assess pupils for symmetry and reactivity to light; asymmetrically dilated pupil in unconscious athlete indicates transtentorial herniation; hyperventilate patient and transport immediately to medical facility

4. Evaluate athlete for other injuries, including skull fracture if scalp integrity disrupted; signs of basilar skull fracture: postarticular hematoma (Battle's sign), rhinorrhea, otorrhea, periorbital ecchymosis (raccoon eyes), and hematotympanum

5. If athlete has remained conscious or rapidly regained consciousness and if cervical spine injury ruled out, take to sideline for observation and re-evaluation

    a. Determine orientation to time, person, and place and presence of amnesia and confusion; observe gait

    b. Asymptomatic athlete has no headache, confusion, dizziness, impaired orientation, impaired concentration, or memory dysfunction either at rest or on exertion

    c. Athlete with persistent symptoms should not return to play

    d. Transport athlete who develops seizures, focal neurologic signs, or deterioration in mental status to medical facility immediately

POSTCONCUSSION SYNDROME

1. Diagnose when symptoms (eg, headache, dizziness, irritability, fatigue, impaired memory and concentration, and slow decision making) persist for days to months
2. Some symptoms aggravated by exercise
3. Perform CT or MRI to exclude intracranial lesions
4. No specific treatment other than rest
5. Use neuropsychiatric tests to monitor recovery
6. Do not allow athlete with postconcussion syndrome to return to competition until all symptoms resolve, both at rest and during exertion

SECOND-IMPACT SYNDROME

    Rapid brain swelling (often fatal) from second mild head injury while still symptomatic from first head injury

PREVENTION OF HEAD INJURIES

1. Athletes in certain contact sports (eg, football, boxing, lacrosse, ice hockey) should wear protective headgear
2. Type and condition of helmets

    a. Pneumatic pockets superior to strap-type suspension

b. Should be intact and properly fitted
c. Replace defective helmets
3. Well-fitted mouth guard can also minimize concussions
4. Rules changes (eg, making "spearing" illegal) can help decrease head and neck injuries
5. Strengthening neck muscles may also reduce number and severity of head injuries

FACIAL TRAUMA

Facial injuries are especially common in sports using balls, racquets, and bats, as well as in high-velocity, direct-contact sports (eg, boxing, karate). While there are many types of injuries, most involve the eyes, ears, nose, and teeth.

EYE INJURIES

Certain findings after eye injury require immediate attention and further evaluation (ie, by ophthalmologist):
1. Blurred vision
2. Loss of visual field
3. Sharp stabbing pain
4. Double vision
5. Abnormal extraocular movement
6. Abnormal pupil
7. Cut or penetrating wound of eyelid or eyeball
8. Abnormal visual acuity

Corneal Abrasion

1. Caused by scratch or foreign material in eye
2. Symptoms: tearing, photophobia, and pain
3. Diagnosed with fluorescein-impregnated paper strips. Corneal epithelial defects look
   a. bright green under ordinary light
   b. bright yellow under cobalt blue light
4. Treatment
   a. Apply topical antibiotics and firm sterile pad dressing, provide adequate analgesia, and re-examine every 24 hrs until healing complete
   b. Carefully remove foreign bodies
   c. Do not patch abrasions caused by contact lens to prevent development of infectious keratitis
   d. Never use topical anesthetics because loss of sensation may result in ulcer

Burn of the Eye

1. Generally due to sun exposure, most commonly in water and snow sports, in which ultraviolet light burns conjunctiva; chemical burns less common
2. Most common symptoms: pain and photophobia
3. Treatment
   a. Systemic analgesics and topical corticosteroid for pain relief
   b. Copious water irrigation for chemical burns
   c. No topical antibiotics

Hyphema

1. Collected free blood in anterior chamber of eye; most common intraocular injury associated with sports
2. Presentation
   a. Initially, blood may disperse and appear as haze in anterior chamber
   b. Pupil is irregular (larger) and reacts slowly to light
   c. Blurred vision
3. Treatment
   a. Most hyphemas resolve within few days
   b. Avoid strenuous activity and remain in bed with head of bed elevated
   c. Use topical steroid or cycloplegic to minimize discomfort
   d. Preserve clot with antifibrinolytic agent
   e. Hospitalize and consult with ophthalmologist; rebleeding common 2–5 days after original bleed and 25–35% of patients also have damage to other eye
4. Complications: late glaucoma, cataracts, blood staining of cornea, and rebleeding

Lacerations of the Eye

1. Common sports injuries repaired fairly easily
2. However, three areas require special care and possible consultation:
   a. Lacerations that cross lid margins
   b. Those involving medial third of lid (possibly including lacrimal area)
   c. Corneal lacerations that may → ruptured globe

Subconjunctival Hemorrhage

1. Damage to conjunctival vessel → blood pooling beneath conjunctiva
2. Usually resolves in 10–14 days without treatment
3. Rule out associated injuries, such as ruptured globe

Posterior Segment Injuries

1. Result from blunt trauma: retinal detachment, retinal edema, choroid rupture, and hemorrhage

2. Signs and symptoms: complaint of flashes of light or sensation of shade or curtain being pulled down over eye, decreased pupillary response, or decreased red reflex
3. May be vision threatening and require prompt referral to ophthalmologist

EAR INJURIES

Auricular Hematoma

1. Cauliflower ear results from untreated auricular hematoma (secondary to direct ear trauma) that becomes organized to cause deformity
2. Treatment to prevent deformity includes
   a. Ice
   b. Hematoma aspiration using aseptic technique
   c. Pressure dressing to prevent reaccumulation: collodion splint or cast formed to ear or through-and-through suture using button for compression; leave cast in place for 5–7 days
   d. If open drainage required, administer prophylactic broad-spectrum antibiotic
   e. Athlete should not participate in sports for 24 hrs and should not sleep on affected ear

Otitis Externa (swimmer's ear)

1. Infection caused by bacterial and fungal species
2. Signs and symptoms
   a. Inflammation, pain, pus, and itching
   b. Acute pain, especially after sleeping on that side
   c. Decreased hearing acuity
   d. Drainage
   e. Acute tenderness to movement of pinna or tragus and narrowed, erythematous canal
3. Treatment
   a. Resolves quickly with proper treatment: corticosteroid or colistin sulfate (make sure tympanic membrane intact before using any topical treatment)
   b. For severe cases: 3% boric acid or 5% acetic acid with isopropyl alcohol
   c. Analgesics if pain severe
   d. Athlete may need to stop swimming
4. Preventive Measures
   a. Keep ears dry, avoid water in ears, wear ear plugs, and drain ears of water
   b. Do not use cotton swabs in ear canal
   c. Never let soap or shampoo in ears

d. Consider using aluminum subacetate solution or alcohol drops after swimming to change pH
e. Use baby oil as protective coating

NASAL INJURIES

Epistaxis (nosebleed)

1. In athletes, most nosebleeds secondary to trauma
2. Anterior nosebleeds (90% of epistaxis cases) relatively easy to treat
   a. Ice and compression usually control bleeding
   b. If not, cauterize site with silver nitrate sticks or electrocautery pen
   c. Occasionally gauze packing required to control bleeding
3. Posterior epistaxis usually more severe, with blood draining into throat
   a. For minor epistaxis:
      (1) Elevate head and pack with gauze, inflated Foley catheter, or specially designed nasal catheter, if available
      (2) Once bleeding controlled, apply topical antibiotic
      (3) Do not blow nose for 24 hrs
      (4) Re-examine in 2–3 days to check for septal hematoma (collected blood between septal cartilage and perichondrium)
   b. For major epistaxis:
      (1) Apply 4–10% cocaine for vasoconstriction and lidocaine for anesthesia, with cotton pledgets left in place for 5–10 min
      (2) Pack nose with petroleum jelly or iodoform gauze, beginning posteriorly
      (3) Leave packing in place 72 hrs and avoid physical activity, hot beverages, and showers until packing removed
      (4) Re-examine in 2 wks
      (5) Possible complications: sinusitis, otitis media, obstructed eustachian tube, and pressure necrosis of nasal or nasopharyngeal mucosa
      (6) Profuse bleeding from nasal fracture usually requires reduction and packing

Nasal Fractures

Nasal fractures vary from simple to severe, depending on force and direction of blow; frontal blows tolerated better than lateral ones.
1. Signs of nasal fracture
   a. Epistaxis
   b. Swelling of nasal dorsum
   c. Ecchymosis around eyes
   d. Tenderness
   e. Deformity

    f. Crepitus
    g. Visible fracture on radiograph
2. Examine to
    a. Identify source of epistaxis
    b. Rule out septal hematoma
    c. Treat septal hematoma with drainage for decompression and nasal packing to prevent recurrence
3. Treatment
    a. Adequate reduction as soon as possible; waiting period necessary if ecchymosis and swelling impede fracture identification
    b. Maximum time for reduction: 4 days for children, 10–12 days for adults
    c. Reduce under local or general anesthesia
    d. Use closed reduction to treat children and unilateral fractures of nasal bones without major deviation; keep intranasal splint in place for 7–10 days
    e. Open reduction indicated for significant septal displacement or when maintaining reduction difficult

TOOTH AVULSIONS

1. If re-implanted expeditiously, totally avulsed tooth may survive
2. Rinse tooth in running tap water to remove loose debris, but do not brush or handle root surface
3. During transport to dentist, keep tooth moist in plastic container with whole milk, saliva, or sterile saline solution, and wrapped in gauze pad
4. After re-implantation, avulsed tooth stabilized to adjacent teeth for 1–2 wks
5. Analgesia, tetanus shot, and antibiotics indicated

Chest and Abdominal Injuries

Serious chest and abdominal injuries from blunt trauma are infrequent in sports, but when they do occur, they can be life threatening. The athlete's appearance after such an incident may be misleading. Thus, to adequately assess athlete's condition, perform serial examinations until pain resolves or diagnosis made.

MECHANISMS OF INJURY

Direct Blows: contusions, fractures, and dislocations

Sudden Deceleration: severe shear stresses on internal organs from their attachments

Compressive Forces: ↑ intrathoracic or intra-abdominal pressure and may result in rupture of hollow or air-filled organs or compression and resultant fracture of solid organs

BLUNT CHEST TRAUMA

Soft Tissue Injuries

1. Muscle Contusions
   a. Signs and symptoms
      (1) Well-localized pain exacerbated by motion in involved area
      (2) Tenderness over area of trauma
   b. Treatment
      (1) Apply ice, and possibly compression, for 1st 24–48 hrs after injury
      (2) Apply heat later to help resolve hematoma
2. Disruption of the Pectoralis Major Muscle
   a. Signs and symptoms
      (1) Severe pain radiating to shoulder and upper arm
      (2) Passive abduction and active adduction of arm very painful
      (3) Palpable defect in pectoralis major muscle
      (4) Radiographs may demonstrate absence of pectoralis major muscle shadow
   b. Treatment

        (1) Treat proximal disruptions conservatively
        (2) Surgically repair distal disruptions near musculotendinous junction

3. Breast Contusions in Female Athletes
    a. Signs and symptoms
        (1) Ecchymosis, pain, and unilateral breast enlargement from hematoma
        (2) Later, post-traumatic fat necrosis and mammographic changes mimicking malignancy
    b. Treatment
        (1) Apply ice during 1st 24–48 hrs
        (2) Use binder or brassiere for support
        (3) No competitive activity until swelling and inflammation subside
    c. Contusion of augmented breasts
        (1) May sustain capsular or implant rupture
        (2) With capsular rupture, breast is softer, with concave profile
        (3) With implant rupture, gradual or immediate breast decompression and masses adjacent to breast
        (4) Surgical repair necessary

Fractures

1. Rib Fractures
    a. Usually 5th to 9th ribs at point of impact or at posterior angle of rib (weakest point)
    b. Signs and symptoms
        (1) Significant pain, often pleuritic in nature, and aggravated by movement
        (2) Palpation at fracture site elicits pain
        (3) Shortness of breath, either from pain or from flail chest secondary to multiple rib fractures
    c. Complications: pneumothorax, hemothorax, lung contusion, liver and spleen lacerations, and kidney injury
    d. Fracture of 1st 3 ribs associated with extreme trauma that may result in great vessel or airway injury
    e. Diagnosis
        (1) AP chest radiograph or anterior oblique rib view
        (2) 50% of fractures not visible on radiographs immediately after injury, but may become evident 10–14 days later
        (3) If fracture noted on early radiographs, obtain inspiratory and expiratory films to rule out pneumothorax and hemothorax
    f. Treatment
        (1) Unless pneumothorax or hemothorax present, treatment primarily supportive: rest and analgesics
        (2) Occasionally intercostal blocks used for short-term pain relief

2. Clavicular Fractures
   a. Signs and symptoms
      (1) Anterior chest pain
      (2) Clinically and radiographically, disruption of normal clavicle contour noted
   b. Treatment: figure-of-eight strap
3. Sternal Fractures
   a. Rare and related to violent traumatic forces
   b. Often associated with cardiac contusions
   c. Patient has anterior chest pain

Separations and Dislocations

1. Costochondral Separation ("slipping rib syndrome")
   a. Increased mobility of one or more lower costal cartilages, which allows anterior costal margins to "slip" over one another
   b. Signs and symptoms
      (1) Costal margin pain precipitated by physical exertion and position change
      (2) Palpable deformity
   c. Treatment: rest, ice, and analgesics
2. Sternoclavicular Joint Dislocation
   a. May be difficult to detect clinically
   b. Severe anterior thoracic pain mimics angina or pleuritic pain
   c. Anterior dislocations most common; treatment depends on injury severity
   d. Posterior dislocations
      (1) May be associated with great vessel or airway impingement or disruption and considered medical emergencies
      (2) Transport athlete with arms against chest
      (3) Monitor vital signs en route to medical facility

Pleural Space Injuries

1. Most often associated with pleuritic chest pain and dyspnea
2. Simple Pneumothorax
   a. Signs and symptoms
      (1) Decreased breath sounds, hyperresonance to percussion, and possibly subcutaneous emphysema on affected side
      (2) Best radiographic view: upright expiratory chest film; if not possible, then lateral decubitus chest view with suspected side superior
   b. Treatment depends on size of pneumothorax and degree of symptoms
      (1) Small, asymptomatic pneumothorax: observation and serial chest radiographs
      (2) Large, symptomatic pneumothorax: chest tube for lung re-expansion

3. Tension Pneumothorax
   a. Life-threatening condition can compromise both respiratory and circulatory systems
   b. Signs and symptoms
      (1) Same as those of simple pneumothorax
      (2) Also distended neck veins, tachycardia, respiratory distress, and possibly hypotension
      (3) Upright expiratory chest films: collapsed lung with tracheal and mediastinal shift away from side of pneumothorax
   c. Treatment
      (1) Immediate decompression with 14-gauge needle inserted in 2nd or 3rd intercostal space in midclavicular line
      (2) Insertion of chest tube
4. Hemothorax and Chylothorax
   a. Hemothorax results from laceration or tearing of intercostal or pulmonary vessels; chylothorax from disruption of thoracic duct from shear forces
   b. Respiratory compromise if significant fluid accumulates in pleural space
   Pleural effusion seen on upright chest films; if patient cannot sit upright, obtain lateral decubitus chest film with affected side in dependent position
   c. Circulatory compromise if bleeding into pleural space significant
   d. Treatment
      (1) If respiratory compromise, promptly insert chest tube to drain fluid
      (2) Repair intercostal artery laceration and thoracic duct disruption when patient stable

Parenchymal Injuries

1. Pulmonary Contusion
   a. Nonsegmental areas of interstitial and alveolar hemorrhage produce edema without parenchymal laceration
   b. Large contusions can cause ventilation-perfusion mismatch and respiratory failure
   c. Signs and symptoms
      (1) Rales
      (2) Cough productive of blood-tinged sputum
      (3) Patchy, ill-defined consolidations on chest radiographs within 1 hr of injury
   d. Conservative treatment: bronchodilators, nebulizer treatment, and nasotracheal suctioning
2. Pulmonary Hematoma
   a. Macroscopic accumulation of blood in lung from pulmonary lacerations
   b. Frequently causes respiratory compromise, and in severe cases may require intubation

    c. Large consolidations of fluid in lung parenchyma on chest radiographs immediately after trauma

3. Pulmonary Emboli

    a. Infrequent consequence of blunt trauma to chest

    b. Signs and symptoms

        (1) Tachypnea and tachycardia

        (2) Cyanosis and respiratory failure

        (3) Chest pain uncommon, but may be present

        (4) ABGs usually show $\downarrow$ PaO_2 and oxygen saturation with relatively normal $PaCO_2$

        (5) Definitive finding: mismatch on ventilation-perfusion scan

    c. Treatment

        (1) Administer IV heparin immediately

        (2) Provide oxygen therapy

        (3) Intubate in cases of respiratory failure

Mucosal Tears

1. Found in trachea, bronchi, and esophagus

2. Signs and symptoms

    a. Precordial or substernal chest pain, possibly radiating to shoulders, neck, or back

    b. Chest radiographs show pneumomediastinum with tracheal and bronchial rupture

3. Diagnose tracheal or bronchial ruptures by bronchoscopy

4. Diagnose esophageal ruptures by esophagography with water-soluble contrast medium

Aortic Rupture

1. Most common site of rupture: just distal to left subclavian artery

2. 80–90% of patients do not survive trip to hospital

3. Signs and symptoms

    a. Severe and tearing substernal or back pain

    b. Findings on chest radiographs

        (1) Widened mediastinum at level of aortic arch

        (2) Abnormal contour of aortic knob or descending aorta

        (3) Left mainstem bronchus depression $> 40°$ below horizontal plane

4. Treatment

    a. Infusion of copious amounts of IV fluids, including blood

    b. Immediate surgical repair

Heart Injuries

1. Cardiac Contusion

    a. Injury results in transmural necrosis

    b. Signs and symptoms

        (1) Chest pain

      (2) Nonspecific EKG changes and CPK elevation

      (3) Regional or global depression of ventricular wall motion, ↓ ventricular ejection fraction, cardiac chamber enlargement, and pericardial effusions on echocardiography and radionuclide angiography

  c. Complications

      (1) Most common: cardiac dysrhythmias

      (2) Other life-threatening complications: CHF; pericardial effusion with tamponade; pulmonary thromboembolism; and myocardial, papillary muscle, or valve rupture

2. Coronary Artery Dissection

  a. May be asymptomatic or result in angina or death

  b. Following dissection, coronary artery obstruction ensues, resulting in MI

  c. Typical ischemic changes on EKG

  d. Treatment

      (1) Conservative if patient stable

      (2) For ongoing ischemia, angioplasty or bypass grafting

3. Intraventricular Septal Defects

  a. Diagnostic triad: chest trauma, systolic ejection murmur, and infarct pattern on EKG

      (1) Murmur present immediately in acute defects

      (2) Appearance of murmur delayed in defects that occur several days after trauma

  b. Treatment

      (1) Spontaneous healing with medical management possible

      (2) Persistent or progressive heart failure and pulmonary hypertension indicate need for surgery

  c. Complications and prognosis related to conduction pathway involvement, size of defect, and coexisting cardiac and noncardiac injuries

ABDOMINAL INJURIES

General Presentation

1. Onset of pain may be immediate, insidious, or even hrs after trauma

2. Contusions

  a. Tenderness confined to area of impact and pain aggravated by tensing underlying muscles (no referred pain)

  b. Contusions may be difficult to distinguish from, or may coexist with, intra-abdominal injury

3. Intra-abdominal bleeding

  a. Causes intra-abdominal irritation, but pain often mild

  b. Minimal tenderness

4. Hollow viscus and gland injuries

  a. Result in severe, initially localized pain that eventually spreads to entire abdomen from diffuse peritonitis

    b. Signs of intraperitoneal injury: abdominal rigidity, involuntary abdominal wall spasm, guarding, referred pain, and loss of bowel sounds

    c. Pain aggravated with body movement

5. Serious abdominal injury and hemorrhage

    a. Cool, clammy skin, pallor or cyanosis, ↑ heart rate, ↓ BP, thirst, and mental status changes suggest shock

    b. Immediate treatment

       (1) Place patient in Trendelenburg's position

       (2) Administer IV fluids; no fluids by mouth

       (3) Apply anti-shock garment

       (4) Transport to trauma center

Abdominal Wall Injuries

1. Muscle Contusions

    a. May cause long periods of discomfort, debilitation, and inability to compete

    b. Treatment: rest, ice, and analgesics

2. Rectus Sheath Hematomas

    a. Rapid swelling of abdominal wall may mimic intra-abdominal injury

    b. Cross-lateral abdominal radiograph may show hematoma

    c. Treatment: large hematomas may require evacuation; otherwise, treat with ice, compression, and analgesics

Spleen Injuries

1. Signs and symptoms

    a. Pain: initially left upper quadrant and referred to left shoulder, progressing to diffuse abdominal involvement

    b. Tenderness over 10th, 11th, and 12th ribs

    c. Pulse often rapid, and other signs of shock may follow

2. Treatment

    a. If no signs of continued bleeding or shock, bed rest and observation in medical facility

    b. If surgery necessary, most splenic injuries from sports can be sutured

    c. Splenectomy is last resort; give Pneumovax in case splenectomy becomes necessary

Liver Injuries

1. Signs and symptoms

    a. Right upper quadrant pain later referred to right shoulder or diffuse over entire abdomen

    b. Tenderness over 10th, 11th, and 12th ribs secondary to fracture

    c. Liver contusions may result in subscapular hematomas, but diagnostic peritoneal lavage frequently negative

2. Treatment
   a. If no signs of continued hemorrhage or shock, bed rest and observation in medical facility
   b. Surgery if capsule ruptures or hematoma continues to enlarge (as seen on CT scans)

Pancreas Injuries

1. Signs and symptoms
   a. Severe abdominal or back pain progressing to diffuse abdominal pain with development of peritoneal signs
   b. Reflex ileus
   c. ↑ amylase level on diagnostic peritoneal lavage
   d. ↑ serum amylase and lipase levels 12–24 hrs after injury
   e. Divided pancreas or mass effect on CT
2. Treatment: usually surgery, especially if severe contusion or divided pancreas

Hollow Viscus Injuries

1. Signs and symptoms
   a. Diffuse abdominal pain and tenderness with peritoneal signs
   b. Diagnostic peritoneal lavage positive for amylase, food, bilirubin, or organisms (bacteria) on Gram stain
   c. Free air on abdominal radiographs and CT
2. Treatment: primary repair of injured structure, except colon injuries, which may require diverting colostomy

Retroperitoneal Injuries

1. Retroperitoneal Hematomas
   a. Signs and symptoms
      (1) Pain severity varies
      (2) Hematuria
   b. Diagnose by ultrasonography, CT, or IV pyelography; reserve arteriography for suspected vascular pedicle injuries
   c. Treatment: conservative (ie, observation and analgesics) unless evidence of shock, expanding retroperitoneal hematoma, or extravasation of urine on IV pyelography; monitor hematuria for resolution

Bladder Rupture

1. Rare with blunt abdominal trauma; more frequent with pelvic fracture incurred in vehicular sports
2. Diagnose by cystography
3. Treatment
   a. Treat small retroperitoneal lesions with Foley catheter or suprapubic cystostomy
   b. Treat intraperitoneal lesions surgically

6

Dermatologic and Infectious Diseases

BACTERIAL SKIN INFECTIONS

Impetigo

1. Highly contagious disorder spread by skin-to-skin contact or by fomites from mats, equipment, or towels
2. Group A β-hemolytic Streptococcus produces crusted, yellowish, weeping lesions around mouth and nose
3. S. aureus produces blisters (bullous impetigo)
4. Treatment
   a. Local debridement of lesions
   b. 10-day course of topical mupirocin ointment t.i.d. or oral antibiotics (erythromycin, penicillinase-resistant penicillin, or cephalosporin)
   c. No sports activities until all lesions resolved

Furunculosis

1. Localized staphylococcal abscess of epidermis in areas of friction (eg, axillae, groin, and buttocks)
2. Treatment
   a. Usually resolves in several days with warm compresses
   b. Occasionally, oral erythromycin or penicillin derivatives for 10 days required
   c. No participation in close-contact sports until lesions dry and resolving

Pitted Keratolysis

1. Superficial infection of weight-bearing surfaces of feet that mimics tinea pedis
2. Circular pits and longitudinal furrows on skin surface
3. Lesions common in long-distance runners, basketball players, and tennis players who have hyperhidrosis and wear occlusive footwear
4. Treatment: frequent changes of footwear and socks, twice daily ap-

51

plication of drying agents, such as 20% aluminum chloride (Drysol) and 5% benzoyl peroxide gel in 3% topical erythromycin (Benzamycin)

VIRAL SKIN INFECTIONS

Herpes Simplex Virus

1. Highly contagious and spread by direct contact
2. Early treatment of herpes-related conditions
   a. Drying agents (5–10% benzoyl peroxide gel, Campho-Phenique, 4% zinc solutions)
   b. Topical acyclovir q3 hrs, 6 times/day, for 7 days applied with finger cot or rubber glove
3. Treatment of initial herpetic lesions
   a. Either 200 mg acyclovir PO 5 times/day or 400 mg t.i.d. for 7–10 days
   b. No participation until lesions dry and resolved for at least 3 days prior to competition
4. Athletes who experience more than 6 recurrences/yr can take 400 mg PO b.i.d. routinely while training and competing

Molluscum Contagiosum

1. Single or multiple pearly, umbilicated, dome-shaped papules containing poxvirus
2. Spread by direct inoculation: wrestlers most often affected
3. Treatment
   a. Curettage quickest and most reliable treatment; resume activity 2–3 days later
   b. Other options: cryosurgery with liquid nitrogen, tretinoin, salicylic acid, and laser surgery

Verrucae Vulgaris (common warts)

1. Epidermal papillomavirus tumors found on plantar surface of feet (transmitted from pool decks and shower rooms) and palms of hand (transmitted from weight apparatus)
2. Paring of wart with scalpel exposes pinpoint black dots (thrombosed capillaries)
3. Treatment
   a. During season: daily applications of keratolytic agents, such as 16% salicylic acid with 16% lactic acid (Duofilm), 40% salicylic acid plaster (Mediplast), or 17% salicylic acid OTC (Compound W)
   b. After season: cryosurgery with liquid nitrogen

FUNGAL SKIN INFECTIONS

Dermatophytes (ringworm fungi)

1. Include tinea pedis (''athlete's foot''), tinea cruris (''jock itch''), tinea corporis (body ringworm), tinea capitis (scalp ringworm), and onychomycosis (nail ringworm)
2. Spread by direct contact from person to person and through moist environments (eg, locker room floors and showers, and shoes)
3. Treatment
   a. Drying agents (Burow's solution), OTC topical antifungal powders and creams, such as miconazole (Micatin), undecylenic acid (Desenex), and clotrimazole (Lotrimin, Mycelex)
   b. Prescription agents: econazole (Spectazole) and ketoconazole (Nizoral)
   c. For resistant cases of onychomycosis: oral griseofulvin 250–1000 mg/day for several months; infrequently, remove toenail

SKIN INFESTATIONS

Pediculosis (''crabs'' or ''lice'')

1. Spread in sporting events by direct contact and in dressing rooms through towels, clothing, and brushes
2. Diagnosed by presence of pruritus without rash and visualization of nits (eggs) on hair follicles
3. Treatment: lindane (Kwell), permethrin (Nix), pyrethrine (RID), and alathion (Ovide)

Scabies

1. Highly contagious mites produce erythematous burrows with tiny papules and vesicles in finger web spaces, axillae, and about waist, ankles, soles of feet, and genitals
2. Diagnosed by microscopic identification of mites
3. Treatment
   a. Topical lindane applied 1 time/week for 2 consecutive wks; participate day after treatment
   b. Wash clothing in hot, soapy water and store for 7–10 days

ENVIRONMENTAL DAMAGE TO THE SKIN

Sunburn

1. Develops 2–6 hrs after skin exposure to ultraviolet B light and produces mild erythema with secondary vesicle formation
2. Prevention
   a. Sunscreen with solar protection factor (SPF) based on skin type

b. Avoid peak exposure hrs (11am-3pm)

c. Cover skin with light, loose, cotton garments

3. Treatment (based on degree of sunburn): cool compresses, topical corticosteroids, oral NSAIDs, and for severe cases, oral corticosteroids

FROSTNIP AND FROSTBITE: SEE CHAPTER 3

TRAUMATIC SKIN INJURIES

Blisters

1. Caused by frictional forces producing intraepidermal skin split, allowing serum accumulation between layers

2. Preventive Measures

a. Properly fitted shoes, talcum-powdered socks, and nylon hose

b. Apply benzoin to harden epidermis over areas of maximum pressure

c. Decrease friction by lubricating with emollients containing urea, lactic acid, mineral oil, glycerin, or petrolatum

3. Treatment

a. Drain large, tense blisters using small needle and leaving roof as protective layer

b. Apply topical antibiotics and occlusive dressing to promote epithelialization

Calluses

1. Hyperkeratosis commonly develops over metatarsal and metacarpal heads in gymnastics, dancing, running, and racquet sports; rowers develop calluses on skin over ischial tuberosity of buttock

2. Can become tender and painful

3. Treatment

a. Pare with scalpel blade and sand with pumice stone after hydration

b. Apply topical salicylic acid or lactic acid nightly

Corns

1. Small, painful, keratinized lesions: either soft lesion between toes or lesion with hard, central, translucent core overlying bony prominence

2. Treatment

a. Properly fitted, padded shoes restore normal function to foot

b. Pare after hydration

c. Apply salicylic acid plaster

Black Heel

1. Asymptomatic black dots or streaks on posterior or lateral heel from rupture of papillary dermal capillaries and extravasation of heme into epidermis

2. Common in basketball, tennis, and racquetball players who routinely make sudden, forceful movements of feet
3. Prevention: fitted heel cups, moleskin, or shoe padding
4. Treatment: none; lesions resolve spontaneously over time

Black Toe (tennis toe)

1. Subungual hematoma, most common under 1st or 2nd toenail, secondary to sudden or repeated trauma
2. Prevention
   a. Properly fitted shoes
   b. Metatarsal pads to plantar flex toes
   c. Re-lace shoes during sporting event
3. Treatment: to relieve pain, puncture nail plate with large-bore needle or wire cautery

Jogger's Nipple

1. Abrasion of nipple and areola from friction of coarse cotton fabric
2. Treatment: wear semisynthetic fabric or silk and apply petrolatum ointment or tape over nipples

Athlete's Nodules

1. Dermal proliferations of collagen from repeated trauma
2. Seen on feet and knees of surfers and on knuckles of boxers
3. Treatment: protective padding, intralesional injection of corticosteroids, and surgical excision

INFECTIOUS DISEASES

Upper Respiratory Tract Infections (URIs)

1. Moderate training may enhance resistance to URIs, but long-distance running (eg, marathon racing) may actually increase susceptibility
2. Associated fever
   a. ↑ cardiac output, oxygen consumption, and lactate production during exercise
   b. ↓ strength, aerobic power, endurance, coordination, and concentration
   c. Places athlete at risk for more serious sequelae (eg, viral myocarditis)

Infectious Mononucleosis

1. Signs and symptoms
   a. Insidious onset with malaise, headache, and fatigue
   b. Splenomegaly in 45% of patients and hepatomegaly in 35%
2. Clinical course

a. Lasts 2–8 months; rarely, can take several months to regain preinfection level of performance
b. Low prevalence of splenic rupture; enlarged spleens may rupture from trauma 4–21 days after symptoms appear

3. Treatment
    a. Permit daily activities within limits (no contact activities); allows for more rapid recovery than complete bed rest
    b. Resume training at 3–4 weeks at modest level and upgrade, allowing 2 days rehab for every day of rest
    c. Treat superimposed infections (occur in up to $\frac{1}{3}$ of patients) appropriately
    d. No corticosteroids unless life-threatening sequelae (eg, airway obstruction, thrombocytopenia, or neurologic problems) occur

Viral Hepatitis

1. Hepatitis A
    a. Most common acute viral hepatitis in young athletes
    b. Transmitted primarily by fecal or oral route; thus, food- and waterborne outbreaks occur
    c. Common prodromal symptoms: fever, nausea, vomiting, abdominal pain, and anorexia
    d. Treatment
        (1) Give immune globulin ASAP after exposure, preferably within 2 wks
        (2) Rest until acute symptoms (ie, fever, nausea, vomiting) subside
        (3) Return to activity individualized for competitive athletes
        (4) Healthy diet and no alcohol
        (5) No Vitamin K unless prothrombin time becomes significantly prolonged

2. Hepatitis B
    a. Transmitted by IV drug use, prenatal spread, sexual activity, and exposure to infected blood
    b. Athletes in close contact with a person with active, acute infection may be passively immunized with hepatitis B immunoglobulin, followed by hepatitis B vaccine
    c. Again, resumption of competitive training determined by individual athlete's response, return of enzyme levels to normal, and response to exercise
    d. Persons with active infection may not participate in certain sports (eg, wrestling): transmission can occur through percutaneous or mucosal contact with infected body fluids

Human Immunodeficiency Virus (HIV) Infection

1. HIV transmission via sport contact remains only theoretical risk; in sports in which bleeding and skin abrasions common (eg, wrestling, boxing, football), no transmission reported to date

2. Occupational HIV exposure is small, but significant risk to health care workers in sports medicine
3. Use gloves when contact with body fluids possible, and use bleach on all surfaces and equipment that may be contaminated with blood
4. Decision for HIV-infected person to continue competitive activities must be individualized, based on discussion and communication with athlete, trainer, physician, coach, and family
5. HIV-positive athletes should avoid extremely strenuous activity, but moderate aerobic exercise may be of benefit

TRAVEL AND INFECTIOUS DISEASE

Diarrhea

1. Up to 60% of athletes who travel internationally develop diarrhea; usually begins in 1st wk and resolves within 2 days
2. Advise on use of local water and consumption of raw vegetables and salads before arrival
3. Prophylactic therapy
   a. Antibacterial agents not often recommended because of possible allergic reactions and side effects such as photosensitivity
   b. Bismuth silicate 2 tablets q.i.d. can reduce diarrhea
   c. Bottled or boiled water usually safe
   d. Wash hands with soap and water before peeling and eating fruit

Immunizations

1. Tetanus booster every 10 yrs following primary series maintains immunity
2. Use tetanus immune globulin only for "dirty" wounds and those for which history of injury and treatment incomplete or unknown
3. Review measles vaccination, as sporadic outbreaks of measles have occurred at athletic events
4. Influenza vaccine
   a. Not recommended for healthy athletes
   b. May consider for athletes in close contact in fall or winter sports to minimize season disruption by infection

Diabetes and Asthma in Athletes

DIABETES MELLITUS

Type I Diabetes

1. Affects younger people and requires insulin therapy
2. Many Type I diabetics active in sports and athletics

Type II Diabetes

1. Appears in middle age or later
2. Often associated with obesity; manageable with proper diet and exercise alone or in combination with oral hypoglycemic medication

Role of Exercise and Effect on Athletic Competition

1. Exercise may benefit health, either as preventive or by improving disease control
2. Diabetic athletes have been prominent in almost every sport: baseball, football, hockey, golf, etc
3. Diabetic under good metabolic control can train essentially same as nondiabetic
   a. May need blood glucose monitoring to ensure control
   b. May need urine monitoring for ketones at times to check for ketonuria
   c. Athlete must know warning signs of high and low blood sugar and ketoacidosis

MANAGEMENT OF DIABETES

1. Achieve prolonged tight blood glucose control by combining medical management, proper diet, and regular exercise
2. Medical management
   a. Type I: combination of short-acting (regular) insulin and intermediate- to long-acting (NPH) insulin
   b. Type II: diet, weight loss, and exercise, and sometimes oral hypoglycemic agent
3. Proper diet

    a. Provides steady blood glucose level; both Type I and II diabetics prone to hypoglycemia

    b. Well-balanced meals consist primarily of carbohydrate, with some protein, and small amount of fat

    c. Afternoon and evening snacks may help prevent hypoglycemia

Benefits of Regular Exercise

1. ↑ muscle sensitivity to insulin and may ↓ insulin production
2. ↑ uptake and utilization of glucose, thus ↓ blood glucose level
   a. Effect more pronounced in insulin-treated diabetics and occurs only if therapy satisfactory
   b. For poorly regulated ketotic diabetics, exercise accentuates hyperglycemia and may ↑ ketonuria, particularly with prolonged exercise
3. **Longterm benefits: weight loss, ↓ risk of cardiovascular disease, ↑ insulin sensitivity, and improved regulation of blood glucose**
4. Physical trainability and performance probably optimized when blood glucose level stable
5. Endurance training ↑ fat utilization, ↑ muscle and liver glycogen stores (allowing much longer activity before supplemental carbohydrate needed), and ↓ blood glucose uptake (↓ likelihood of hypoglycemia)
6. Good blood glucose control facilitates muscle mass development

Contraindications to Exercise

1. Exercise EKG warranted if
   a. Patient older than 30–40 yrs
   b. Duration of diabetes exceeds 10–25 yrs
   c. Symptomatic atherosclerotic disease present
   d. Other primary risk factors for cardiovascular disease present
2. Diabetics with peripheral neuropathy or microangiopathy should
   a. Avoid exercises that traumatize feet; substitute swimming and cycling for walking and jogging
   b. Examine feet daily and keep nails carefully trimmed
   c. Wear properly fitted shoes and socks to minimize blisters, corns, and calluses
   d. Periodically file calluses with pumice stone
   e. Treat foot injuries immediately to prevent complications
3. Diabetics with proliferative retinopathy
   a. Precluded from strenuous or jarring activities (eg, weight lifting and contact sports, gymnastics, and running) and any activity that ↑ heart rate dramatically and ↑ systolic BP over 180 mm Hg
   b. Precluded from scuba diving and exercise while inverted (eg, some yoga positions, headstands).

EXERCISE GUIDELINES

1. Establish good blood glucose control before starting exercise program

2. Measure blood glucose levels before, during, and after exercising
3. Pregame anxiety may mimic hypoglycemia, causing athlete to take inappropriate steps that lead to hyperglycemia, resulting in accentuated ketoacidosis or poor performance
4. Before competing, experiment with altering insulin and food intake and then exercise under conditions similar to competition (eg, same time and similar energy expenditure)
5. ↑ intensity and duration of activity in slow, progressive fashion
6. In hours before exercising, ingest slowly absorbed carbohydrates to maintain adequate blood glucose levels
7. Exercising within 1 hr of injecting regular insulin (or 2½ hrs of injecting intermediate insulin) speeds absorption and ↓ time to peak effect; to prevent this
   a. Avoid exercise, if possible, when insulin effect peaks
   b. Alter injection site (eg, thigh, gluteal area, abdomen, triceps, shoulder) depending on exercise activity, injecting at site that will not be exercising intensively
   c. If exercise commonly done soon after injection of regular insulin, may need no alteration
8. ↑ body temperature ↑ rate of insulin absorption; thus, warm-up duration and amount of clothing worn should be reasonably consistent if exercise occurs within 1st hr after injecting regular insulin
9. Extra medication or ↓ food intake may be needed on days of ↓ activity
10. ↓ medication or ↑ food intake may be appropriate on days of ↑ training duration or intensity
11. When exercise lasts several hours (eg, marathons and other endurance events), Type I diabetics should
    a. ↓ basal dose of insulin by as much as 50%
    b. Consume supplemental food (about 60 kcal) every 30–45 min
    c. Closely monitor blood glucose
12. Medication requirements ↓ in early months of training (10–40% ↓ typical) and remain lower as long as training continues
13. Every modification of insulin dose and every change in nutritional status requires evaluating effects of those changes on exercise and performance

Avoiding Hypoglycemia Associated with Exercise

1. Early symptoms of "insulin reaction" or hypoglycemia
   a. Fatigue
   b. Weakness
   c. Tremor
   d. Headache
   e. Hunger
   f. Numbness or tingling of lips or extremities
2. Signs that others (eg, coaches, other athletes) should know

    a. Staggering gait

    b. Slurred speech

    c. Clumsy movements (eg, dropping or spilling things)

    d. ↓ Performance

    e. Confusion

    f. Irritability

3. Measure blood glucose before exercise and have food readily available for supplemental feeding.

   a. If preactivity blood glucose level <100 mg/dl, eat pre-exercise snack

   b. If preactivity level >100 mg/dl, may need small snack after activity

   c. If preactivity level >250 mg/dl, avoid exercise until urine ketone value negative

4. Hypoglycemia more likely to occur during evening exercise and less likely in morning

   a. Thus, avoid exercising in evening, or if exercise cannot be avoided, expect possible hypoglycemia at night and next day, and

       (1) ↓ amount of insulin that peaks after eating and during eating
       or

       (2) Consume more food before (light carbohydrate meal 2 hrs before event) and possibly after exercise

       (3) Eat carbohydrate-rich diet to restore glycogen to pre-exercise levels within 24 hrs

   b. Diabetics who exercise early in morning should take part of daily insulin as long-lasting insulin evening before or take fraction (25–50%) of usual dose 2½-3 hrs before exercise

5. During and after exercise, hypoglycemia more common and more severe in tightly controlled diabetics and in those with Type I diabetes longer than 10 yrs

6. ↓ insulin that peaks during exercise when hypoglycemia occurs with such activity

7. Short-acting insulin, normally taken before meal, might not be needed on days of activity; more insulin might be required on non-training days

8. Emergency Measures

   a. Subcutaneous or IM injection of 1 mg of glucagon ↑ blood glucose level within min

   b. Keep glucagon emergency kit or sugar (preferably both) available

   c. Instruct someone on site (other than diabetic) in administering medication

CLEARANCE FOR SPORTS

1. Stable diabetes control prior to participation: glucose levels of 60–300 mg/dl with no evidence of ketosis

2. No evidence of diabetic complications
3. Cautious trial of training and competition before full clearance for participation
4. Blood glucose control easier in continuous, progressive, steady, aerobic sports than those requiring short, explosive bursts of energy
5. No absolute contraindication to participation in high-risk sports (eg, scuba diving, skydiving, mountaineering, hang-gliding, etc.) or endurance events in extremely cold weather, but athlete and family should be informed of risks and advised of appropriate precautionary measures

EXERCISE-INDUCED ASTHMA

Exercise-induced asthma is more common in children, but affects persons of all ages and is very rarely life-threatening.

Onset

1. Triggered by respiratory water loss and airway cooling during exercise
2. Typically athlete must ↑ heart rate to 170 bpm and maintain for 5-8 min to trigger episode

Presentation

1. Bronchospasm usually begins 10–15 min after exercise and subsides spontaneously within 30–60 min ("early response")
2. Then refractory period of 30–90 min, when further exercise does not lead to recurrent bronchospasm
3. Some have second bronchospasm 4–12 hrs later ("late response")
4. Severity varies with duration and intensity of exercise
5. Prolonged exercise may actually result in less bronchospasm than moderate workouts, so athlete may be able to "run through" symptoms
6. Severity also affected by environmental conditions and underlying lung disease

Diagnosis

1. Consider exercise-induced asthma in athletes who present with postexertional cough, chest tightness, shortness of breath, fatigue, or postexertional nasal congestion
2. Children may have cough or stomach ache
3. Confirm diagnosis by
   a. Pulmonary function testing before and after exercise
   b. Methacholine challenge test to establish bronchial hypersensitivity
   c. Successful therapeutic trial with inhaled β-agonist in patients with characteristic history

4. Further studies may be indicated to search for exacerbating factors (eg, allergies or infections)

Initial Management to Reduce Symptoms

1. Judicious use of exercise
2. Short bursts of exercise → reflex bronchodilation; trained athletes exhibit exercise-induced bronchodilation > sedentary persons
3. Training effect also ↑ VO_2max, work capacity at given heart rate, and maximum voluntary ventilation, and ↓ heart rate at given workload

Preventive Measures

1. Athlete may benefit from
   a. Choosing less ''asthmagenic'' sport
     (1) Short bursts of activity followed by rest (eg, golf, baseball, tennis, weight training)
     (2) Sport performed in warm, humid environment (eg, swimming, water polo)
   b. Position within given sport (eg, soccer goalie)
   c. Geographic location (eg, Florida vs Minnesota)
2. During workouts, breathe slowly through nose and avoid hyperventilation
3. Avoid allergens and environmental irritants before and during exercise
4. In cold, dry environments, wear mask or scarf over mouth and nose to reduce symptoms
5. Warm up 45–60 min before event to take advantage of postbronchospasm refractory period

PHARMACEUTICAL OPTIONS FOR CONTROLLING THE DISEASE

1. First-choice drug: inhaled β-agonist 10–15 min before exercising that can also be used to reduce postexercise symptoms; oral β-agonists less useful because of delayed action and ↑ side effects
2. Inhaled cromolyn sodium 10–20 min before exercise; not useful for ↓ current symptoms, but helpful for athletes who do not respond to or who cannot tolerate side effects of β-agonists; may combine cromolyn and β-agonists
3. Other medications
   a. Theophylline: partially effective, but side effects limit use
   b. Antihistamines: generally ineffective, though some patients benefit
   c. Anticholinergic drugs (eg, inhaled ipratropium): may limit symptoms, but not prophylactic
   d. Topical decongestant: may ↓ exercise-induced nasal congestion

    e. Corticosteroids (inhaled or systemic): little use in exercise-induced asthma

    f. Calcium channel blockers: may benefit, but longterm use not yet thoroughly studied

4. International Olympic Committee allows theophylline, cromolyn, and selected β-agonists; most athletic organizations require advance written notice of athlete using β-agonist to control exercise-induced asthma

Cardiac Problems

HYPERTROPHIC CARDIOMYOPATHY (HCM)

HCM, the most common cause of sudden and unexpected death in athletes, is a disease of cardiac muscle associated with hypertrophic left ventricle and areas of myocardial fiber disarray.

Presentation

1. Usually no symptoms or only mild ones
2. Sudden death uncommon in asymptomatic or mildly symptomatic adult patients; sudden death in mild cases more likely in preadolescent children
3. Most common symptom: dyspnea, followed by angina pectoris, fatigue, presyncope, and syncope, also palpitations and dizziness; exercise may exacerbate symptoms
4. Syncope is ominous; disqualify any athlete with HCM and syncope from participation in strenuous sports

Auscultatory Findings

1. Left ventricular lift, prominent 4th heart sound, and harsh, crescendo-descendo systolic murmur
2. In some, a thrill
3. More blowing holosystolic murmur at apex and radiating toward axilla, signifying mitral regurgitation
4. Maneuvers that ↓ preload (eg, Valsalva's maneuver, standing posture, amyl nitrite) ↑ gradient and murmur
5. Maneuvers that ↑ preload (eg, squatting) ↓ gradient and murmur

LEFT VENTRICULAR HYPERTROPHY (LVH)—ATHLETE'S HEART SYNDROME

If athlete has only mild LVH, normal diastolic function, and no symptoms, risk for sudden death presumed to be very low

CORONARY ARTERY ABNORMALITIES

Anomalous Origin of a Major Coronary Artery

1. Sudden death during exercise noted in athletes
   a. Whose left main coronary artery originated from right coronary sinus
   b. Whose right coronary artery originated from left coronary sinus
2. Cause of death unclear, but assumed to be acute take-off angle of anomalous artery, which is stretched, compressed between great vessels, or otherwise traumatized

Coronary Atherosclerosis

1. In athletes over 30, coronary atherosclerosis causes 90% of sudden deaths
2. Sudden death: first clinical manifestation of CAD in 25% or more of all coronary patients; most athletes who die suddenly from coronary atherosclerosis have no previous symptoms
3. Athlete's history, EKG, and echocardiogram may reveal previously undetected MI; treadmill test may be abnormal

MYOCARDITIS

Myocarditis may be acute or chronic; usually viral in North America, but also caused by drugs, lead, catecholamines, and allergens

Pathophysiology

1. Myocardial involvement may be focal or diffuse, but lesions randomly distributed in heart; clinical effects depend on location, size, and number of lesions
2. Viral carditis may damage conducting system or be focal (myocardial) and result in predisposition to arrhythmias
3. Risk of potentially lethal arrhythmias not linked to acute phase of disease

Clinical Presentation

1. Clinical manifestations: range from asymptomatic state to fulminant CHF
2. In most cases, myocarditis self-limited and unrecognized

Diagnosis

1. Physical examination: normal unless left ventricular dysfunction significant
2. Suspect myocarditis
   a. When EKG shows focal or generalized left or right ventricular dysfunction

b. If athlete develops dysrhythmias or conduction disturbances and has no other evidence of underlying heart disease
c. With prolonged respiratory tract infection or marked unexplained ↓ in exercise tolerance

MITRAL VALVE PROLAPSE (MVP)

MVP, common finding in athletes, manifested by ↑ mitral valve leaflet area; mitral valve thickened and myxomatous transformation often present

Symptoms

1. Most persons with MVP asymptomatic
2. Symptoms attributed to MVP include
   a. Atypical chest pain, usually sharp, left precordial, that is either fleeting or lasts several hrs (more common in women); usually unrelated to physical activity
   b. Dyspnea, fatigue, dizziness, and palpitations

Diagnosis by Auscultation

1. MVP hallmark: nonejection systolic click moving earlier in systole when sitting than when standing
2. Varying degrees of mitral regurgitation (systolic murmur)

Complications from MVP

1. Infectious endocarditis
2. Supraventricular and ventricular dysrhythmias
3. Transient ischemic attacks
4. Partial strokes
5. Sudden death (extremely rare)

PARTICIPATION IN ATHLETICS

1. Totally asymptomatic persons with no family history of premature death may participate if no evidence of Marfan's syndrome or significant mitral regurgitation
2. Bethesda Conference recommends disqualifying athletes with MVP from strenuous athletic competition in presence of
   a. History of syncope
   b. Family history of sudden death due to MVP
   c. Disabling chest pain or chest pain worsened by exercise
   d. Complex ventricular arrhythmias
   e. Significant mitral regurgitation with moderate or marked cardiomegaly
   f. Marfan's syndrome associated with MVP

CARDIAC EVALUATION OF ATHLETES

Auscultation

1. Provides clue to hypertrophic cardiomyopathy, valvular heart disease, Marfan's syndrome, arrhythmias, or myocarditis
   a. Hypertrophic cardiomyopathy: see section on HCM
   b. Marfan's syndrome: aortic diastolic murmur, systolic ejection sound, systolic murmur (either left sternal border or mitral area), and loud 2nd heart sound
   c. Mitral valve prolapse: see section on MVP
2. Distinguishing causes of systolic ejection murmurs
   a. Pay particular attention to 2nd heart sound and timing of aortic and pulmonary valve closures
   b. Most common murmur: soft midsystolic murmur not associated with any cardiac abnormality (innocent or functional murmur in 30% of young athletes)
   c. Provocation maneuvers (Valsalva's, standing, squatting, amyl nitrite inhalation) can help distinguish causes
   d. If suspect diagnosis other than functional murmur, perform EKG and echocardiography

Electrocardiography

1. Sinus bradycardia common in athletes and considered normal, particularly in aerobic or endurance athletes
2. Other normal variant EKG abnormalities in athletes listed in Table 8–1.
3. Arrhythmias common to athletes (ie, sinus arrhythmia, bradycardia, junctional rhythm, premature atrial contractions) disappear with exertion, are considered benign, and require no special followup
4. EKG changes suggestive of LVH more frequent in athletes

Table 8–1. Electrocardiographic Abnormalities That May Be Normal Variants in Athletes

Sinus bradycardia
Intermittent junctional rhythm
First-degree heart block
Mobitz-I second-degree heart block (Wenckebach's phenomenon)
Incomplete right bundle branch block
Nonspecific T-wave changes
Minor ST segment depression or elevation
Occasional atrial premature and ventricular premature contractions on 24-hour Holter monitoring

Echocardiography

1. Most reliable test to detect HCM, CV manifestations of Marfan's syndrome, myocarditis, MVP, previous MIs, congenital heart anomalies, other valve abnormalities, and some coronary artery anomalies
2. However, it is costly, time-consuming, and presents problem of whether asymptomatic athlete with demonstrated abnormality should be disqualified from participation
3. "Quick look" (parasternal, long-axis, and short-axis views) with color flow Doppler screening can reduce costs

Treadmill Testing

1. Main indication for exercise testing of athlete: to rule out CAD
2. Criteria for testing athletes
   a. Age older than 35 yrs and high risk for cardiac events
   b. Symptoms: chest discomfort with exertion, unusual dyspnea, dizziness, lightheadedness, syncope, or palpitations
   c. Known CV disease
   d. Abnormal cardiac findings that may indicate risk for athletic participation
3. Withhold from competition athlete with positive treadmill test for ischemia until disease ruled out
4. Do not disqualify asymptomatic athlete based on single positive treadmill test without further studies

Holter Monitoring

1. Indicated for athletes with history of syncope
2. Monitor athletes while they practice their sport

Loop Electrocardiographic Recorder (Event Recording)

1. Used for longterm monitoring
2. More likely to identify syncopal episodes than Holter monitoring

Upright Tilt Table Testing

1. Diagnostic standard when athlete has unexplained syncope and no structural heart disease
2. Neurocardiogenic syncope (mediated by vagus nerve) most common cause

Spine Injuries

STINGERS AND BURNERS

Mechanism of Injury

1. Impact of head, neck, and shoulder with another athlete, playing surface (Fig. 9–1), or another fixed object (common in football)
2. Results in
   a. Shoulder depression while cervical spine hyperextended, hyperflexed, or laterally flexed to opposite side
   b. Brachial plexus stretching on affected side
   c. Injury to upper trunk of brachial plexus or C5-C6 nerve roots
3. Although symptoms may be same, underlying injury can be quite different in severity and affect either brachial plexus or nerve root

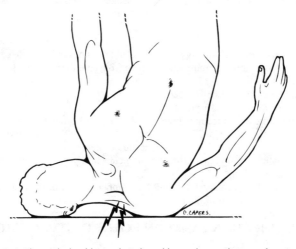

Fig. 9–1. The neck-shoulder angle is forced beyond normal range of motion by shoulder depression with cervical hyperextension and lateral bending toward the contralateral shoulder.

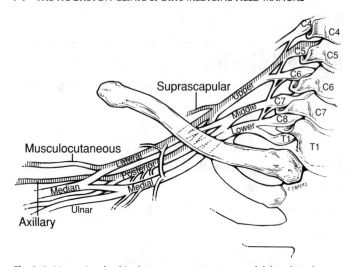

Fig. 9–2. Nerves involved in the most common patterns of delayed weakness after traction injury to the brachial plexus. The weak muscles allow the clinician to track the site of injury: C5, rhomboid minor and major; C5–6, supraspinatus and infraspinatus (suprascapular nerve), coracobrachialis, biceps, and brachialis (musculocutaneous nerve), deltoid and teres minor (axillary nerve), and serratus anterior (long thoracic nerve). Very often, the serratus anterior is spared, which indicates that the injury is distal to this point.

Symptoms

1. Severe burning, stinging paresthesia, and weakness of variable severity in one upper extremity that radiate from shoulder distally through arm to fingers
   a. Paresthesia lasts few sec to few min
   b. Weakness for 15 min or longer
2. Paresthesia and accompanying weakness (most often of upper trunk brachial plexus C5-C6-innervated muscles: shoulder abductors, external rotators, and elbow flexors) due to neural injury (Fig. 9–2)
3. Unilateral symptoms most often indicate injury no more proximal than nerve root
4. Bilateral syndromes (affecting both upper extremities) most often due to spinal cord injury

CLASSIFICATION BASED ON EXTENT OF DAMAGE TO NEURAL ELEMENTS

1. Transient Neuropraxia: No structural damage; paresthesia and weakness resolve in min; soreness and bruising about shoulder and supra-

clavicular triangle (Erb's point) may persist for days, during which Tinel's sign can be elicited

2. Neurapraxia: Numbness resolves in min, but some muscle weakness lasts up to 6 wks
3. Axonotmesis: Weakness even after compliance with 6 wks of rehab program
4. Neurotmesis: Extensive injury results in continued residual weakness despite 6 mos of rehab

Spectrum of Injuries Associated with Stingers or Burners

1. Single transient nerve irritation with no residual deficits
2. Those that recur as many as 50 times during season without residual
3. Complete nerve root avulsion at spinal cord level results in catastrophic permanent anatomic and functional deficits to upper extremity

EVALUATION AND TREATMENT

1. At time of symptoms
   a. Player removes as much of uniform and protective gear as possible to allow inspection of cervical spine, shoulders, and arms.
   b. Test
      (1) Active ROM of cervical spine and upper extremities
      (2) Manual muscle strength of both upper extremities
      (3) Gross sensation to light touch in dermatomes C5-T1
      (4) Biceps, triceps, and brachioradialis reflexes
   c. If all findings normal and pain resolved, player can return to game once protective gear checked and modified with additional shoulder padding and neck roll
   d. While on sidelines, immediately ice any area of tenderness to minimize bruising; check for recurrent symptoms
2. Immediately after competition
   a. Re-evaluate with same tests done on field, but in greater detail
   b. If supraclavicular triangle palpation soreness only symptom, use ice pack for up to 72 hrs and then apply heat
   c. Promptly refer any athlete with ↓ cervical spine motion, pain, and radicular symptoms for imaging studies to rule out vertebral or disc injury
   d. No contact sports until re-examination ensures that no weakness has developed
3. Before exposure to further contact
   a. Goal: to prevent recurrent injury, because subsequent injuries tend to be more severe
   b. Evaluate again for ROM, strength, sensation, and reflexes
   c. If any weakness detectable (representing nerve injury), restrict exposure to further injury until weakness resolves

    d. Once increasing strength evident, begin conservative weight training program until strength is = bilaterally

    e. Modify shoulder pads to decrease shoulder depression and cervical deviation

    f. Further evaluate unresolved weakness, sensory changes, or recurrent stingers, and forbid further contact sports

Preventive Measures

1. Use high-quality shoulder pads to absorb compression forces
2. Following stinger or burner, additional padding to shoulder pads and neck roll helpful

Rehabilitation

1. ROM and light stretching exercises help regain full pain-free cervical spine and affected shoulder ROM
2. Then start slowly progressive strengthening exercise program to build up neck and scapular stabilizing muscles
3. Continue strengthening exercises during season and offseason to prevent recurrence

CERVICAL INJURIES

Mechanism of Injury

1. Cervical injuries with associated neurologic trauma caused by hyperflexion plus axial loading
2. Leading cause of cervical spine injuries in football: direct axial loading from initial contact with helmet crown
3. Most cervical spine injuries due to compressive flexion
    a. Compressive failure of anterior vertebral column demonstrated by ↓ anterior column height
    b. Lateral radiographs provide best view (Fig. 9–3); AP view can show vertical fracture line (''crush cleavage'' injury)
4. Vertical compression is other common mechanism of injury
    a. Symmetric failure of both anterior and middle columns results in symmetric ↓ cervical vertebral body height
    b. Lateral radiographs reveal
        (1) Superior or inferior endplate concavity of involved vertebra
        (2) Bone retropulsion into canal as force vector ↑
5. Higher stages of compression flexion injuries may produce chronic instability from ligamentous disruption posteriorly, but most axial-loading vertical compressive injuries do not

Screening Criteria

1. Obtain lateral cervical spine view
2. Consider future problems when

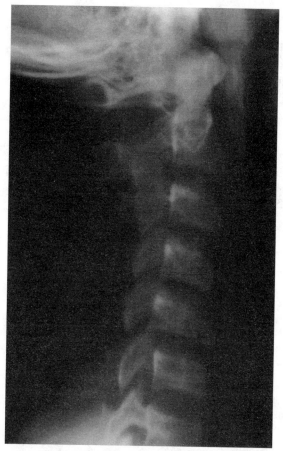

Fig. 9–3. Lateral radiograph shows a compressive flexion injury of C5.

    a. Radiographic evidence of instability exists
    b. Spinal canal measures < 10 mm from posterior vertebral body
       of C5 to spinolaminar line
3. No participation in contact sports with mobile os odontoideum
4. No participation with history of fractures involving 2 columns, cervical fusion, or decompression: excessive stress placed on adjacent intervertebral motion segment
5. Assess cervical spinous process avulsion fractures or compression injuries involving < 20% of anterior vertebral body height for insta-

bility on flexion and extension lateral cervical spine radiographs; athlete with stable spine can play with minimal risk to cervical region

Cervical Strains

1. Most frequent cervical injuries to athletes: traumatic strains to cervical paraspinal muscles
2. More frequent in muscles that span more than one joint
3. Occur when cervical paraspinal muscles are overloaded eccentrically
   a. High-intensity forceful contraction in eccentric mode increases muscle soreness
   b. Weakness and fatigue predispose muscle to injury-producing loads; proper warm-up helps reduce muscle injuries
4. Often, precipitating event not apparent to injured athlete; symptoms may peak 24 hrs after trauma
5. Treatment
   a. Ice, NSAIDs, and cervical flexibility and strengthening exercises
   b. Short-term immobilization (when needed) of injured muscle in lengthened position may ↓ reinjury susceptibility
6. Strain injuries often recur because of poor rehab practices

Cervical Sprains

1. Injury to cervical spine ligamentous structures
2. May present same as strain, but more severe injuries (Grade III) can involve cervical subluxation or frank dislocation, with catastrophic neurologic sequelae
3. More commonly, injuries consist of partial tears (Grade I and II injuries)
   a. ↓ cervical motion
   b. No neurologic sequelae
4. Lateral cervical radiographs with flexion and extension views needed to evaluate patients with persistent symptoms
5. Treatment: immobilization, rest, NSAIDs, and cervical ROM and strengthening exercises

ON-FIELD EVALUATION

1. Athlete who can walk alone or with assistance off playing field
   a. Is immediately assessed for residual sensory or motor deficits on sidelines
   b. Undergoes thorough examination in locker room
   c. Must have radiographic examination before resuming contact activities
   d. May return to play if symptoms resolve and ROM full
2. If athlete remains down on field, rule out unstable cervical spine injury before moving player
   a. Establish or maintain adequate airway

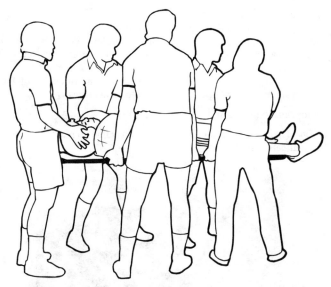

Fig. 9–4. Technique for transport off the field.

    b. If prone, log roll athlete, clear mouth, and perform neurologic examination

    c. Question athlete about pain, tingling, numbness, blackouts, or dizziness, and assess memory to check for closed head injury

    d. Presume any athlete with neck and arm pain or findings suggesting closed head injury has unstable cervical spine injury until proven otherwise

Transportation Off Field

1. If evidence of cervical tenderness or abnormal neurologic findings, properly transport player off field
2. Maintain head control during transport
3. If backboard available, log roll player onto it and 5 people (2 on each side, 1 at head) transport athlete off field (Fig. 9–4); do not remove helmet on field
4. Lacking backboard, position 2 people on either side at shoulders and waist and 1 each at feet and head; carriers lock arms under supine player, and person controlling head grasps posterior head and neck with hands

OFF-FIELD EVALUATION

1. Once patient on sidelines or in locker room, perform more detailed examination

2. Contraindications to return to play
   a. Arm numbness, tingling, weakness, or pain
   b. Persistent, painful, limited ROM or neurologic deficit
   c. Restricted cervical ROM with pain, which often indicates occult, potentially catastrophic injury
   d. With lower extremity findings, restrict play until full radiographic evaluation completed, even if symptoms later resolve

Radiographic Evaluation

1. Take lateral cervical spine radiograph with helmet in place if physical examination findings abnormal

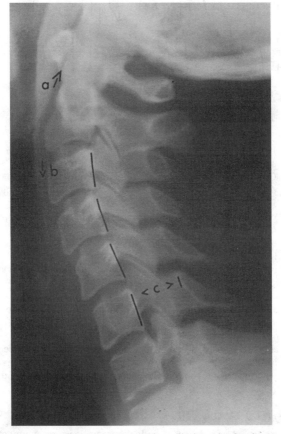

Fig. 9–5. Normal lateral cervical spine radiograph shows landmarks: (a), pre-dens interval; (b), convex curve; (c) sagittal diameter of the spinal canal.

   a. Visualize and meticulously inspect all 7 cervical vertebrae (Fig. 9–5)

   b. Seek both obvious and subtle signs of injury

   c. Prevertebral or retropharyngeal soft-tissue shadow may be only clue to cervical spine injury; shadow should be ≤ 4 mm directly anterior to C3 vertebral body

   d. Posterior vertebral bodies and spinolaminar line should be continuous

2. If lateral radiograph normal, remove helmet and perform full examination

3. Obtain remaining trauma series radiographs: AP, open-mouthed, and oblique views

4. After evaluating these views, obtain flexion and extension lateral views

   a. Pre-dens interval > 3 mm on flexion view suggests C1-C2 instability

   b. Available spinal cord space of < 13 mm suggests dens fracture

   c. Any difference in angulation > 11° or translation > 3.5 mm suggests instability

5. If no abnormality noted, but patient has neurologic or radicular findings, obtain MRI

FRACTURES OF THE THORACIC AND LUMBAR SPINE

Fractures of the Transverse or Posterior Spinous Processes

1. Are stable injuries
2. Isolated transverse process fractures may be 2° to torsional injury
3. Isolated posterior spinous process fractures may result from flexion injury
4. Pain due to associated soft tissue injury
5. No cast or brace needed; ↓ activity sufficient
6. Fractures from hyperflexion or torsional injury may be associated with significant ligamentous injury and instability and require long-term immobilization or surgery

Compression Fractures

1. Result from axial loading of spine
2. Disruption of anterior vertebral body and variable injury to posterior ligamentous complex
3. Based on physical examination and plain radiographs, determine stability and treatment options

   a. Carefully palpate posterior spinous processes and interspinous ligament

   b. If step-off significant or interspinous interval markedly painful, posterior ligamentous injury present; treat with molded hyperextension brace or cast

   c. If no posterior ligamentous injury, treat with thoracolumbar corset or hyperextension brace

   d. Compression fractures associated with loss of > 50% anterior vertebral cortex height on plain radiographs unstable and often require surgical stabilization in addition to brace or cast

Burst Fractures and Fracture-Dislocations

1. Injury to anterior and posterior vertebral body and posterior ligamentous complex
2. Severe, unstable injuries that commonly require surgical treatment

SPONDYLOLYSIS AND SPONDYLOLISTHESIS

   Spondylolysis: defect in vertebral posterior arch

   Spondylolisthesis: forward subluxation of vertebral body from loss of posterior spine stabilization.

MECHANISM OF INJURY AND ASSOCIATION WITH CERTAIN SPORTS ACTIVITIES

1. Repetitive lumbar spine flexion and extension activities
2. Pars interarticularis lesions occur in > 20% of female gymnasts and disproportionately affect adolescents who participate in diving, weight lifting, football, wrestling, high jumping, and rowing

Symptoms

1. Low back pain
   a. Usually localized to low back, but may be referred to buttock and posterior thigh
   b. Rarely radiates below knee and into calf and foot
   c. Exacerbated with activities and partially relieved with rest
2. Hamstring tightness: ↓ flexibility and inability to bend and touch toes
3. Symptoms may be from specific traumatic event or of insidious onset

Physical Examination Findings

1. Spondylolisthesis: paravertebral muscle spasm, hamstring tightness, and palpable step-off in posterior spinous processes
2. Usually no neurologic symptoms
3. List to one side when standing

Radiographic Findings

1. Lateral view demonstrates any vertebral body forward subluxation
2. Oblique views: show defects in pars interarticularis
3. However, plain radiographs cannot rule out possibility of developing stress fracture

4. For early diagnosis, obtain technetium bone scan to detect stress injury or CT to detect fracture

Treatment of Spondylolysis

1. Symptomatic spondylolysis rare
2. Treat symptomatic adolescents with bed rest, physical activity reduction, and molded body brace
3. Complete symptom resolution usually takes 8–12 wks
4. Once symptoms resolve, adequately reconditioned athlete may return to all activities
5. Persistently symptomatic athlete may need spinal fusion

Treatment of Spondylolisthesis

1. Depends on severity of symptoms and degree of vertebral body slippage
2. Treat symptomatic athletes with ≤ 33% subluxation with activity restriction and molded lumbosacral brace
    a. Once symptoms resolve, athlete may start reconditioning program and return to all activities, including contact sports
    b. Follow with serial lumbosacral radiographs every 6 months, or sooner if low back symptoms recur
3. Adolescent athletes with ≥ 33% subluxation or those who show progression of slippage may require surgical treatment, even if asymptomatic
4. Persistently or recurrently symptomatic athletes may require surgery

Fractures and Dislocations about the Shoulder

CLAVICULAR FRACTURES

Classification

1. By pattern (greenstick, oblique, transverse, or comminuted) or by anatomic site
2. Clavicular fractures in children
   a. Most nondisplaced or minimally angulated greenstick fractures
   b. Commonly result from fall on shoulder point or outstretched hand
3. Clavicular fractures in adults
   a. Often displaced and overriding
   b. Most result from fall on outstretched hand
   c. In hockey and lacrosse, often caused by direct blow to clavicle

Clinical Presentation in Older Children and Adults

1. Crepitus, swelling, and tenderness
2. Athlete holds involved extremity to ↓ pain

Radiographic Evaluation

1. Routine AP view of clavicle
2. 45° cephalic tilt view

NONSURGICAL TREATMENT

1. Immobilization for comfort
2. Sling and ice for nondisplaced fracture
3. Figure-of-eight harness to reduce displaced fracture

SURGICAL TREATMENT INDICATED

1. Debridement of open fracture
2. Neurovascular compromise unresolved with closed reduction
3. Several irreducible, displaced fragments

4. Mediastinal compression associated with posteriorly displaced medial clavicular fracture

FRACTURES OF THE DISTAL THIRD OF THE CLAVICLE (FIG. 10–1)

1. Type I
   a. Occur between acromioclavicular (AC) and coracoclavicular (CC) ligaments
   b. Stable and require only sling

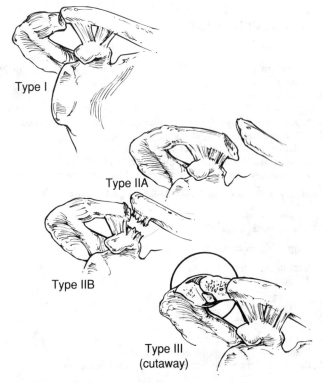

Fig. 10–1. Distal clavicle fractures. Type I occur between the acromioclavicular joint and the coracoacromial ligaments. The intact ligaments hold the fragments in place. Type IIA fractures occur medial to the coracoacromial ligaments. Type IIB fractures involve a tear of the coracoacromial ligaments. Type III involve only the articular surface of the clavicle.

2. Type II
   a. Occur medial to or through CC ligaments
   b. Unstable and often require surgical stabilization
3. Type III
   a. Involve distal clavicle articular surface
   b. Often missed and present with late sequelae
4. Document solid bone union before athlete returns to activity

Possible Associated Injuries

1. Rib fractures
2. Pneumothorax or hemothorax
3. Tears in trachea or main bronchi
4. Neurovascular injuries

Possible Complications

1. Nonunion (rare, but serious) often 2° to inadequate immobilization
2. Malunion (functional or cosmetic problem) can be corrected by osteotomy, internal fixation, or bone grafting
3. Post-traumatic arthritis may occur at clavicular articulations

SCAPULAR BODY, ACROMION, AND CORACOID FRACTURES

Scapular Fractures

1. Classification by anatomic site
   a. Type I: fractures of scapular body
   b. Type II: fractures of apophysis, including coracoid and acromion
   c. Type III: fractures of superior lateral angle, including neck and glenoid
2. Classification by site and degree of injury
   a. Class I: coracoid and acromion fractures and small fractures of scapular body
   b. Class II: glenoid and neck fractures
   c. Class III: major scapular fractures

Mechanism of Injury

1. Scapular neck fracture: direct trauma or fall on shoulder point or outstretched arm (axial loading)
2. Scapular body fracture: direct trauma, often with high energy
   a. In adults, significant trauma required to fracture scapula
   b. Sudden muscle contraction may contribute to fracture fragment displacement
3. Acromion fracture: direct superior blow
   a. Fracture line typically lateral to AC joint and minimal displacement occurs

    b. Acromion may also fracture from axial loading with humeral
       head
4. Coracoid fracture
    a. Isolated, as from direct blow to coracoid during sporting event
    b. Or associated with AC dislocation while CC ligaments remain
       intact; AC joint injury not uncommon in adolescent athletes and
       associated coracoid fracture must be ruled out

Clinical Presentation

1. Scapular Fracture
    a. Arm held adducted and protected from movement; abduction ex-
       tremely painful
    b. Local tenderness, ecchymosis, and hematoma
    c. Deep inspiratory pain
2. Acromion Fracture
    a. Pain on attempted arm abduction
    b. Flattened shoulder, localized pain, swelling, and tenderness
3. Coracoid Fracture
    a. Local pain, tenderness, pain on shoulder adduction and elbow
       flexion, and deep inspiratory pain
    b. Severely displaced coracoid fragments may be palpable close to
       axillary fold
    c. Neurologic deficits may result from fractured coracoid contusing
       brachial plexus cords

Radiographic Evaluation

1. AP shoulder view, tangential oblique scapular view, and axillary
   view
2. In younger athletes, contralateral shoulder joint plain films may help
   in evaluation
3. Tangential and AP views may demonstrate scapular body or neck
   fracture
4. Confirm acromial fractures on AP and axillary lateral shoulder views
5. Assess acromial fractures in young athletes with 30° caudal tilt and
   supraspinatus outlet views
6. Axillary lateral view essential if coracoid fracture suspected
7. Stryker notch and Goldberg's posterior oblique 20° cephalic tilt views
   may also visualize coracoid fracture
8. In selected cases, CT may be helpful for defining fracture

Treatment

1. Scapular Fracture
    a. Indications for surgical fixation in athlete rare
    b. Reduction of most scapular neck fractures and restoration of gle-
       noid to anatomic position not necessary; sling may immobilize
       shoulder for comfort

    c. Scapular body fracture usually does not require surgery because surrounding muscles provide excellent healing environment; pain management important during healing

2. Acromion Fracture
   a. Nondisplaced fractures respond well to symptomatic treatment and sling immobilization
   b. Some orthopedists prefer tension band wire for fixation of displaced fractures

3. Coracoid Fracture
   a. Isolated fractures need no specific treatment because anatomic alignment not essential for adequate healing and future athletic competition
   b. Open reduction may be indicated if displacement significant or if complete 3rd degree AC separation combined with significantly displaced coracoid fracture
   c. Early exploration of possible suprascapular nerve or brachial plexus entrapment may be needed to avoid future complications

POSSIBLE ASSOCIATED INJURIES

1. Scapular fracture: rib fractures, pneumothorax, pulmonary contusion, clavicle fracture, spine damage, and neurovascular damage
2. Rotator cuff disruption: fractures of acromion and scapula
3. Loss of shoulder function and anatomic symmetry; bone irregularities may cause soft tissue impingement on ribs and result in pain, crepitus, and limitation of motion

Glenoid Fractures

Classifications in Adults (Fig. 10–2)
1. Type I: avulsion of anterior margin
2. Type II: glenoid fossa transverse fracture with inferior triangular fragment displaced with humeral head
3. Type III: oblique glenoid fracture exiting at midsuperior scapular border and often associated with AC fracture or dislocation
4. Type IV: horizontal fracture exiting through medial border of body
5. Type V: Type IV plus fracture separating inferior half of glenoid

Classification in Young Athletes
1. Those associated with glenohumeral joint dislocation
2. Those extending from scapular neck fractures (often comminuted)

Mechanism of Injury

1. During sporting events, direct forces produce injury (Fig. 10–3)
2. Type I: frequently occurs with shoulder dislocations and subluxations
   a. Posterior dislocation may result in posterior rim glenoid fracture

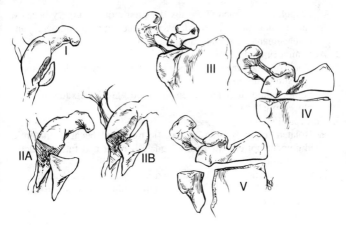

Fig. 10–2. Ideberg's classification of intra-articular fractures of the glenoid.

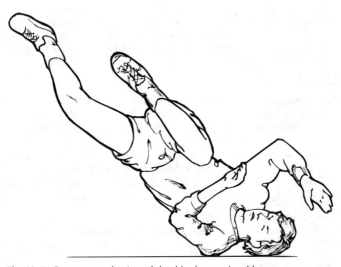

Fig. 10–3. Common mechanism of shoulder fracture in athletes.

    b. Anterior dislocation may knock off glenoid fragment, with or without avulsion force from surrounding capsular structure

3. Type V: typically results from violent shoulder trauma

Radiographic Evaluation

1. AP, tangential scapular lateral, and axillary lateral radiographs
2. CT: helpful in determining fragment size and humeral head position

Treatment

1. Large, displaced glenoid fragment may need open reduction with screw fixation
2. Aggressive surgical repair of displaced glenoid fragments indicated to avoid recurrent instability
3. Open reduction and fixation of Type I fracture may obviate reconstruction with fragment fixation or bone graft
4. Indications for surgical management of Type II through V fractures less clear
5. Follow large anterior glenoid fracture treated nonsurgically with frequent radiographs and physical examinations to assess fracture healing and joint stability
6. Treat adolescent athlete with minimally displaced fracture conservatively
7. Treat older children with 1 cm or larger fragments like adults, with fragment replacement plus anterior shoulder reconstruction

Possible Associated Injuries

1. Clavicle fracture
2. Pneumothorax
3. Rib fractures
4. Spine damage
5. Shoulder dislocation
6. Brachial plexus injury
7. Neurovascular damage

    Possible Complication: shoulder instability that impedes future athletic competitiveness

PROXIMAL HUMERAL FRACTURES

Types of Fractures

1. Displaced: when separation between fragments more than 1cm or fragment angulated more than 45° from other fragments; displaced fracture may have 2, 3, or 4 parts
2. Head-splitting proximal humerus fractures (usually tuberosities or surgical neck)
3. Dislocations of fractured bones

Mechanism of Injury

1. Athlete abducts, extends, and externally rotates arm to break fall
2. Falling directly on lateral shoulder
3. Falling on outstretched hand

Clinical Presentation

1. Pain, swelling, tenderness, and dysfunction about shoulder
2. Crepitus and local ecchymosis, latter occurring 24–48 hrs after injury

Radiographic Evaluation: trauma series

Treatment

1. Most minimally displaced and managed with initial immobilization and early ROM
2. For 2- or 3-part fractures, ORIF
3. Children with proximal humeral fractures rarely require surgery

Possible Complications

1. Avascular necrosis, brachial plexus injury, myositis ossificans, "frozen" shoulder, infection, pneumothorax, hemothorax, nonunion, and malunion
2. Hardware failure
3. Growth deformity in children ranges from small loss of motion to limb length inequalities and angular deformity

SOFT TISSUE INJURY TO THE ACROMIOCLAVICULAR (AC) JOINT

Mechanism of Injury

1. Most common: direct trauma, especially fall onto shoulder point
2. Acromion driven downward, rupturing ligaments

Classification (Fig. 10–4)

1. Type I: incomplete AC ligament tear; CC ligament and deltoid and trapezius muscles remain intact
2. Type II: complete AC joint disruption, but not complete separation of joint surfaces; CC ligament and deltoid and trapezius muscles remain essentially intact
3. Type III: complete AC and CC ligament tears; some detachment of deltoid and trapezius muscles from scapula
4. Type IV: Type III injury in which clavicle dislocates posteriorly instead of superiorly
5. Type V: severe form of Type III with extensive disruption of deltoid and trapezius muscles

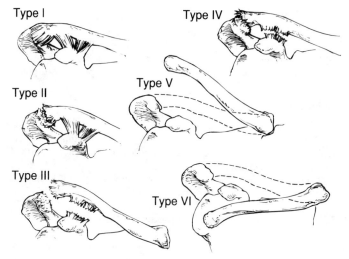

Fig. 10–4. Classification of acromioclavicular injuries. Type I, the acromioclavicular and coracoclavicular ligaments are not disrupted. Type II, acromioclavicular ligament disrupted, but the coracoclavicular ligament is intact. Type III, both acromioclavicular and coracoclavicular ligaments are disrupted. Type IV, both ligaments are disrupted and the distal end of the clavicle is displaced posteriorly. Type V, both ligaments are disrupted and the muscles are detached. Type VI, both ligaments are disrupted, and the end of the clavicle is dislocated inferiorly.

6. Type VI: complete AC and CC ligament disruptions with inferior clavicle dislocation

Clinical Presentation

1. Type I: only sign may be AC joint point tenderness; joint remains stable, with only mild discomfort at extremes of motion
2. Type II: more AC joint tenderness and moderate swelling; may be some joint laxity and slight step-off between acromion and clavicle
3. Type III: more tenderness and swelling, with pain and ↓ motion; clavicle displaced superiorly relative to acromion
4. Type IV: same as Type III, but clavicle displaced posteriorly or posterosuperiorly
5. Type V: distal clavicle displaced superiorly, occasionally with skin tenting
6. Type VI: may be severe swelling and associated neurologic or vascular injuries; acromion prominent because clavicle displaced inferiorly

Radiographic Evaluation

1. AP shoulder view with beam at 15° cephalic inclination
2. Stress views can distinguish Type II injury from Type III; take with 10–15 lbs weight tied to wrist, not held in hand
3. Axillary or Alexander's lateral view to check for posterior displacement

Radiographic Findings

1. Type I: normal radiographs
2. Type II: slight clavicle elevation and AC joint widening
3. Type III: clavicle displaced superiorly and CC distance 25–100% greater than normal
4. Type IV: clavicle displaced posteriorly on axillary or Alexander's lateral view; may be slight elevation on AP view, with AC joint widening
5. Type V: clavicle displaced superiorly and CC distance 100–300% > normal
6. Type VI: clavicle displaced inferior to acromion or coracoid process

Treatment

1. Type I
   a. Rest injured joint initially in sling
   b. Ice and analgesics lessen discomfort
   c. As symptoms ↓, active ROM and resume sports as tolerated
2. Type II
   a. Treat nonsurgically
   b. One conservative option accepts any displacement and uses sling followed by early ROM
   c. Another option uses device (e.g., Kenny Howard sling) to hold reduced clavicle in position; however, significant amount of continuous force over distal clavicle for several wks may cause skin ulcers under shoulder strap
   d. Resume sports when ROM full and painless
   e. Place protective pad on top of contact athlete's shoulder to prevent pain and additional ligament injury
3. Type III–VI
   a. Many orthopaedists recommend conservative treatment
   b. Hughston Clinic treats Type III (and IV, V, and VI) injuries with ORIF unless some contraindicating complications or patient does not want surgery
      (1) Repetitive activity may result in dull shoulder and neck ache from residual joint instability when Type III treated conservatively
      (2) Resultant malfunction rarely allows athlete to return to throwing sports

(3) Myriad surgical techniques available for repairing AC dislocations

Late Complications

1. Type II subluxations: frequent recurring pain due to restraint of unstable joint; instability may result in arthritis
2. Type III dislocations treated nonsurgically: fatigue, aching, and soreness in shoulder and neck muscles with excessive use; complaints of comparative weakness, unsightly deformity, and inability to excel in throwing sports and archery
3. Late complications, pain, and arthritis minimal when Type III dislocations treated nonsurgically

SOFT TISSUE INJURIES TO THE STERNOCLAVICULAR (SC) JOINT

Mechanism of Injury

1. Most common: indirect force
   a. Posteriorly directed force to anterolateral shoulder may cause anterior SC joint instability
   b. Anteriorly directed force to posterolateral shoulder may cause posterior SC joint instability
2. Direct force (e.g., posteriorly directed force to anteromedial clavicle) can dislocate SC joint

Classification

1. Based on anterior or posterior position of displaced clavicle
2. Anterior dislocations more common
3. Injury may result in SC joint sprain, subluxation, or dislocation

Clinical Presentation

1. Arm held adducted and internally rotated
2. Mild, moderate, or severe pain, depending on degree of displacement
3. Variable amount of swelling may obscure deformity
4. In anterior dislocations, medial clavicle can be quite prominent
5. In posterior dislocations, normal inner clavicle prominence lost; swallowing or breathing may be difficult if esophagus or trachea compressed

Radiographic Evaluation

1. Routine radiographs difficult to interpret
2. 40° cephalic tilt radiograph can help
3. CT: best imaging technique for diagnosing SC joint subluxation or dislocation

Treatment

1. Sprain
   a. Ice for 12–24 hrs and sling immobilization for few days
   b. ROM as tolerated
   c. When full, painless ROM regained, resume sports (usually within 1–2 wks)
2. Subluxation
   a. Figure-of-eight clavicle strap to reduce SC joint or sling until pain subsides
   b. ROM as tolerated
   c. Allow noncontact sports when full, painless ROM restored
   d. Allow contact sports 6–8 wks after injury
3. Acute Anterior Dislocation
   a. Reduction, while easy, usually unstable and joint redisplaces
   b. Some surgeons accept deformity and do not attempt reduction
   c. Most, however, recommend closed reduction and immobilization with figure-of-eight clavicle strap for 4–6 wks
   d. If redisplacement occurs after traction released, place arm in sling for 2 wks, then ROM exercises as tolerated
   e. Cosmetic deformity may persist, but seldom interferes with function
   f. Open reduction seldom indicated; closed reduction and percutaneous pin fixation never indicated
   g. Resume sports based on same criteria for subluxations
4. Acute Posterior Dislocation
   a. First direct attention to any mediastinal injury; neurovascular, tracheal, or esophageal compression require consultation
   b. Posterior dislocations usually stable and reduced as anterior dislocations, but with anterior force
   c. Sooner closed reduction attempted, easier it is to perform; after 48 hrs, closed reduction seldom possible
   d. If closed reduction unsuccessful, open reduction necessary because of risk of compression of mediastinal structures
   e. After reduction, immobilize shoulder in figure-of-eight clavicle strap or spica cast for 4–6 wks
   f. No contact sports for additional 6–8 wks
   g. Late complications rare

Shoulder Instability

FUNCTIONAL ANATOMY OF THE SHOULDER

Static stabilizers: glenoid, labrum, glenohumeral (GH) ligaments, and coracohumeral ligaments

Dynamic stabilizers: rotator cuff, subscapularis, and long head of biceps

Instability may result if any of these stabilizers are deficient

Changes Associated with Instability

1. Tearing of interior labrum (most visible arthroscopic change) from shearing loads of humeral head as it translocates
2. Bankart lesion: detachment of thickened anterior inferior quadrant where inferior GH ligament attaches
3. Hill-Sachs lesion: compression fracture of posterior humeral head
4. Stretching of middle GH ligament
5. Stretching or tearing of inferior GH ligament
6. Superior labral tears at biceps attachment
7. Rotator cuff tears
8. Changes in articular surface

Classification Criteria

Direction

1. Location of humeral head in reference to glenoid
2. Can be anterior (most common), posterior (relatively rare), inferior, or multidirectional

Causes of Instability

1. Can be traumatic (eg, previous primary dislocation) or cumulative result of repetitive microtraumatic events (eg, pitching)
2. Can also be atraumatic (eg, hyperplastic, hyperlax persons with instability)

   Degree of Instability: Frank dislocation or varying amounts of joint subluxation

   Patient Control: Are events voluntary and controlled, or involuntary in occurrence?

TWO GENERAL GROUPS OF INSTABILITY

1. TUBS: Traumatic, Unidirectional instability with Bankart lesions or ruptures of GH ligaments at glenoid rim that require Surgery
2. AMBRI: Atraumatic, Multidirectional instability that is Bilateral, with Rehabilitation treatment of choice, but if surgery necessary, Inferior capsular shift is done

ACUTE GLENOHUMERAL INSTABILITY

Mechanism of Injury

1. Anterior Dislocation: occurs when arm abducted, extended, and externally rotated
2. Posterior Dislocation: occurs when arm adducted and flexed
3. Violent mechanism of injury (eg, contact during football game) more likely to produce dislocation
4. Noncontact injury (eg, sustained while throwing baseball) more likely to produce subluxation

Clinical Presentation

1. Acute Anterior Dislocation
   a. Very painful shoulder with spasm of surrounding musculature
   b. Arm held externally rotated and slightly abducted
   c. Humeral head palpable in anteriorly dislocated position
   d. May be associated neurovascular (particularly axillary nerve) injury
2. Acute Posterior Dislocation
   a. Arm held internally rotated and adducted across body
   b. Inability to externally rotate arm past $0°$
   c. Palpable posterior prominence
   d. More noticeable coracoid process on dislocated side

Radiographic Evaluation

1. To confirm direction of dislocation, identify associated fractures, and reveal impediments to reduction
2. AP view in scapular plane shows humeral head completely out of socket in anterior dislocation; with posterior dislocation, head may overlap glenoid structures, making recognition difficult
3. Lateral view in scapular plane (Y view) shows humeral head anterior to glenoid in anterior dislocation and vice versa in posterior dislocation
4. Axillary view shows humeral head compression fracture, glenoid rim fracture, and anteriorly or posteriorly dislocated humerus
5. Post-reduction series ensures adequacy of reduction and documents any fractures that may have occurred during reduction

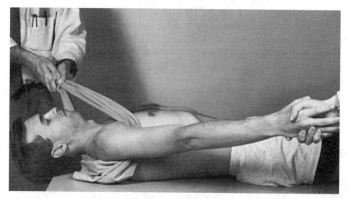

Fig. 11–1. Traction-countertraction reduction maneuver.

Treatment

1. Acute Traumatic Anterior Dislocations
   a. Reduce as quickly and atraumatically as possible; may need pain medication
   b. Abduction/External Rotation Technique
      (1) One of more effective methods on field
      (2) With patient supine or prone, abduct and externally rotate arm and push humeral head back in place (using thumb)
   c. Traction/Countertraction Method (Fig. 11–1)
      (1) Useful if assistant and table available
      (2) Apply longitudinal traction to arm in line with deformity while gently externally rotating arm
      (3) Apply countertraction using sheet wrapped around patient's chest
   d. The Hippocratic Method
      (1) Another useful single-person technique
      (2) With patient supine, apply in-line traction to injured arm using external rotation as needed, while placing foot along chest wall just below—never in—axilla
   e. After Reduction
      (1) Use sling for comfort
      (2) After initial spasms subside within a few days, start circumduction exercises and discard sling
      (3) Use ROM exercises to ↑ abduction and external rotation and strengthen rotator cuff
      (4) On regaining full ROM and strength, allow return to competition; brace that ↓ abduction and external rotation may be used in sports such as football

2. Acute Traumatic Posterior Dislocations
   a. Early reduction and pain relief important
   b. With patient supine, apply traction with arm adducted in line with deformity, using internal rotation as needed while assistant simultaneously applies lateral traction
   c. After reduction
      (1) If joint stable, apply sling and swathe
      (2) If shoulder subluxates or redislocates, use abduction/external rotation brace
      (3) Start wrist and elbow movements immediately, and start ROM and rotator cuff strengthening exercises in stable shoulder when initial discomfort subsides
      (4) Allow return to competition when full ROM and strength return
      (5) No effective brace for posterior dislocations
3. Surgery: may be indicated initially if soft tissue interposition blocks reduction or if significantly displaced tuberosity or glenoid fracture present

Possible Complications

1. Recurrent dislocation: most common complication after anterior dislocation, particularly in younger patients and athletes
2. In young athlete, chance of dislocation that produces unstable shoulder is extremely high
3. Fractures associated with high-energy trauma include
   a. Glenoid rim and humeral head compression fractures (anterior and posterior dislocations)
   b. Greater tuberosity fractures (anterior dislocations)
   c. Lesser tuberosity fractures (posterior dislocations)
4. Surgery may be necessary for acute traumatic dislocations that fail rehabilitation and redislocate

RECURRENT GLENOHUMERAL INSTABILITY

Mechanism of Chronic Injury

1. Humeral head insufficiently contained by normal shoulder restraints.
2. Results in spectrum of disorders
   a. Recurrent frank joint dislocation
   b. Gross humeral head subluxation
   c. Subtle subluxations that, over time, present as shoulder pain and weakness

Clinical Presentation

1. Chronic Anterior Instability
   a. Pain, apprehension, instability, or giving way of shoulder, especially during abduction and external rotation
   b. Anterior or posterior pain

2. Chronic Posterior Instability
   a. Anterior or posterior pain
   b. Reproduce symptoms through adduction, flexion, and internal rotation of arm
3. Chronic Multidirectional Instability
   a. Atraumatic and associated with hypermobility
   b. Component of inferior instability; with symptoms of anterior or posterior instability, there may be pain and clicking when arm is dependent, and sulcus sign
   c. Repetitive microtrauma in hypermobile shoulder with multidirectional instability can create unidirectional (anterior or posterior) instability
   d. Causes more continuous functional disability than does unidirectional instability

Physical Examination

1. General
   a. Look for asymmetry or atrophy of shoulder and musculature
   b. Assess for generalized ligamentous laxity (also evaluate contralateral shoulder and other joints)
   c. Rule out cervical disc disease and radiculopathy
2. Shoulder
   a. Palpate for tenderness
      (1) Rotator cuff and subacromial space may be tender anteriorly, posteriorly, or laterally
      (2) Biceps tendon and glenohumeral interval may be tender, both anteriorly and posteriorly
   b. Assess ROM to evaluate shoulder flexion, abduction, and rotation
   c. Check rotation in both 0° and 90° abduction; in anterior instability, lack of external rotation in abduction secondary to apprehension, but losses up to 20° abduction common
   d. Perform motor examination to assess any weakness and rule out neurogenic cause of shoulder symptoms; pay particular attention to external rotators (ie, rotator cuff) to assess integrity and strength
3. Stress Tests to evaluate joint stability
   a. Load-and-Shift Test (Fig. 11–2)
      (1) Tests for anterior and posterior instability
      (2) Apply force in line with humerus to compress GH joint
      (3) With one hand, cradle GH joint with thumb in front and remaining 4 fingers behind
      (4) Then lever or translate arm anteriorly and posteriorly, back and forth, assessing for "clunk" as humeral head exits glenoid, or for reproduction of symptoms
      (5) Determine zone of instability by varying humeral abduction and adduction

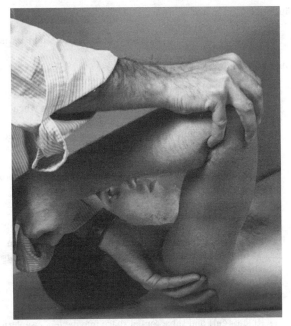

Fig. 11–2. The load-and-shift or "clunk" test.

b. Apprehension Test
   (1) Standard: with arm in 90° abduction and 90° external rotation, push anteriorly on posterior humeral head (Fig. 11–3A)
   (2) Labral: with arm in 130° abduction and 90° external rotation, place one hand posterior to GH joint while grasping elbow with other hand, and push forward on GH joint (Fig. 11–3B)
   (3) Pain occurs if joint unstable and apprehension if prone to recurrent dislocations
c. Relocation Test (Fig. 11–3C)
   (1) Perform in conjunction with apprehension tests
   (2) Posteriorly direct force on humeral head from front
   (3) This resolves pain from apprehension tests, allowing for greater external rotation
d. Sulcus Sign
   (1) Tests for inferior instability
   (2) Apply downward force through humerus while patient sits
   (3) Observe and palpate lateral acromion for opening (sulcus) created by inferior translation of humeral head
   (4) Common in multidirectional instability

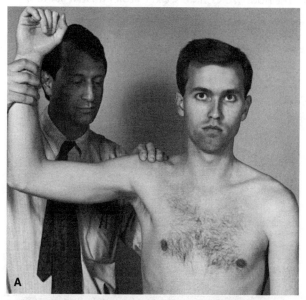

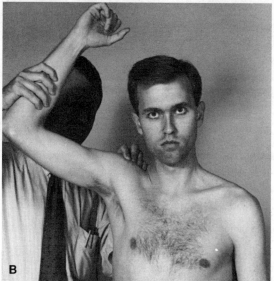

Fig. 11–3A and 11–3B. (A) Standard apprehension test for anterior instability with the arm in 90° of abduction, 90° of external rotation. (B) Labral apprehension sign with the arm at 130° of abduction, 90° of external rotation. The examiner's hands are placed as shown, pushing forward on the humeral head while stabilizing the elbow.

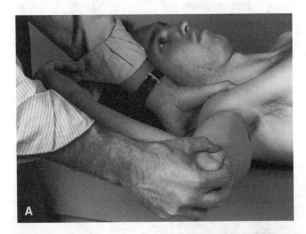

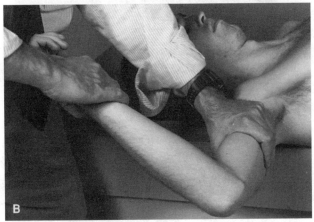

Fig. 11–3C. (A) Apprehension test and (B) relocation test.

Radiographic Evaluation

1. Routine radiographs: AP, axillary, and subacromial outlet views
2. Special views
   a. West Point view: provides tangential view of anterior inferior rim of glenoid and any lesions (eg, Bankart lesion)
   b. Stryker notch view: demonstrates defects in humeral head (eg, Hill-Sachs lesion)
3. CT arthrogram and MRI: reveal further detail of glenoid rim defects, other bony abnormalities, labral damage, and capsular injuries

Treatment

1. Anterior Instability
   a. Treat any inflammation
   b. Then strengthen dynamic shoulder stabilizers, emphasizing subscapularis and infraspinatus of rotator cuff
   c. Treat recurrent dislocations surgically at season's end
   d. Subluxaters may respond to supervised rehab to strengthen dynamic stabilizers; surgically repair those who fail to improve
   e. Surgery directly addresses pathologic structures
      (1) Bankart procedure or similar repairs that ↓ capsular volume eliminate recurrent dislocations, apprehension, and pain, and are excellent for athletes in collision sports
      (2) Throwing athletes require special consideration to preserve external rotation with muscle function
         (a) Arthroscopic reconstruction may be indicated if injury occurs near end of playing season, but longterm results have yet to approach success of open reconstruction
         (b) Jobe's capsulolabral reconstruction technique achieves stability and preserves proprioception and function
   f. Patients with repetitive microtrauma and atraumatic instability
      (1) Usually subluxate rather than dislocate
      (2) Need supervised rehab
      (3) May need arthroscopy to assess and treat secondary damage (eg, labral and rotator cuff tears)
      (4) May need surgery if fail rehab
         (a) Neer's capsular shift technique ↓ capsular volume and tightens attenuated tissues
         (b) Treatment of choice in throwing athletes: Jobe's capsulolabral reconstruction (adequately controls inferior redundancy)
2. Multidirectional Instability
   a. Rehab to stabilize shoulder girdle and strengthen dynamic stabilizers
   b. Strengthen global shoulder to stabilize joint; treating only one component or direction of instability accentuates others
   c. Reserve surgery for those who fail conservative treatment and demonstrate continued impairment, but treat entire problem
3. Posterior Instability
   a. Rehab by strengthening scapular stabilizers and rotator cuff, especially infraspinatus and teres minor
   b. Reserve surgical repair for only most severe cases, as results not encouraging

RETURN TO PLAY

1. Criteria: full ROM, no pain, and adequate shoulder strength
2. Rest may be necessary before strengthening can succeed

3. Wear protective harness to reduce further episodes, although function compromised
4. Change pitchers' positions and swimmers' events as long as symptoms persist
5. After surgery, rest to allow healing, then 4–6 months' rehab before returning to competition
6. Throwing athletes require specific return-to-throw program after rehab
7. Surgery for posterior instability may need 6–12 months' rehab before returning to competition

SUPERIOR LABRUM ANTERIOR POSTERIOR (SLAP) LESIONS OF THE SHOULDER

Types of SLAP Lesions (Fig. 11–4)

1. Type 1: superior labrum fraying
2. Type 2: labrum fraying and separation of labrum from underlying glenoid (most common type)
   a. Type 2a: labrum fraying plus partial separation of labrum from underlying attachment
   b. Type 2b: total separation or avulsion of significant portion of labrum from glenoid
3. Type 3: bucket-handle tear of superior labrum with central displacement of tear; peripheral portions of labrum remain intact
4. Type 4: bucket-handle tear of superior labrum that extends into biceps tendon; biceps tendon and torn labrum can displace into joint space

Associated Injuries

SLAP lesions may occur as isolated tears or in combination with acromioclavicular arthritis, partial or complete rotator cuff tears, and GH instability

Mechanism of Injury

Acute traumatic event: falling on abducted, forward flexed arm; violent throwing event; catching heavy object; or ''jerking'' traction injury

Clinical Presentation

1. Pain with overhead movements in abduction, external rotation, and extension (eg, tennis serve or throwing baseball)
2. Night pain and pain when lifting heavy objects
3. Occasionally, numbness and tingling or history of instability

Physical Examination

1. Positive impingement tests, instability on load-and-shift test, rotator cuff weakness, and positive apprehension testing

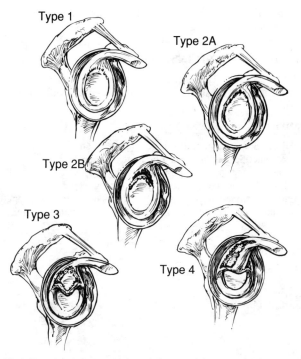

Fig. 11–4. Type 1 lesion (upper left) with fraying of the superior labrum. Type 2a lesion (upper right) with fraying, as in Type 1, together with partial separation of the underlying labrum. Type 2b lesion (center) with separation of the superior labrum from the underlying glenoid. Type 3 lesion (lower left) with a displaced bucket-handle tear that leaves the biceps tendon intact. Type 4 lesion (lower right) with a bucket-handle tear that extends into the biceps tendon.

2. If both apprehension and impingement signs (+)
   a. Use subacromial bupivacaine injection to eradicate impingement sign
   b. Presence of continued positive labral apprehension testing confirms SLAP lesion associated with impingement syndrome

Radiographic Evaluation

1. Reliable imaging of SLAP lesions difficult
2. Obtain AP views in internal and external rotation, axillary view, and Alexander's view
3. CT arthrography may help determine presence and type of SLAP lesion

4. Conventional MRI has not, thus far, reliably distinguished normal variants from pathologic tears

SLAP LESIONS AND INSTABILITY

1. Isolated labrum flap tear can cause functional instability
2. If mechanical instability present, associated instability may cause pain

Treatment

1. All SLAP lesions require surgical intervention
2. Associated lesions must also be treated at surgery
3. After surgery, perform protected Codman exercises for 1–3 wks, followed by active ROM and strengthening exercises
4. Early identification and appropriate treatment result in excellent function and high potential for return to previous levels of activity

Shoulder Impingement and Rotator Cuff Lesions

MECHANISM OF INJURY

Impingement Syndrome

1. Rotator cuff tendons compromised because of repeated abrasion or load (particularly to supraspinatus tendon) beneath coracoacromial arch
2. Outlet impingement occurs when supraspinatus outlet narrowing → mechanical rotator cuff irritation
3. "Critical zone": just medial to supraspinatus tendon insertion site on greater tuberosity
4. Impingement can be 2° to congenital or developmental acromial abnormalities or to previous greater tuberosity fracture
5. Acromioclavicular joint arthritis may narrow supraspinatus outlet and → impingement and rotator cuff lesions
6. Impingement from abnormal scapular mechanics may occur with normal capsule and normal rotator cuff strength, but functionally compromised arch

Rotator Cuff Lesions

1. Primary causes: intratendinous and extratendinous factors
2. Secondary factors: GH instability from cuff injury
3. Overuse injury: from repetitive overhead movements
   a. Repetitive microtrauma to rotator cuff from repetitive overhead motion can cause cuff tendinitis and inflammation
   b. ↓ subacromial space volume potentiates impingement process
4. Major trauma: infrequent cause of rotator cuff tear; most often, minor shoulder trauma extends pre-existing chronic tear, producing sudden, acute pain with more profound weakness
5. GH instability a common cause of impingement syndrome and rotator cuff lesions in young throwing and overhead athletes; direct treatment at underlying shoulder instability

CLASSIFICATION

Impingement

1. Stage I
   a. Edema and hemorrhage
   b. Seen in younger patients, especially those who use arm overhead excessively
2. Stage II
   a. Fibrosis and tendinitis due to mechanical inflammation
   b. Seen in 25- to 40-year-old group
3. Stage III
   a. Rotator cuff tears, biceps lesions, or bony alteration at anterior acromion and greater tuberosity
   b. Seen in older patients

Rotator Cuff Tears

1. Partial Tears: bursal surface tears, articular surface tears, and intratendinous tears (Fig. 12–1)

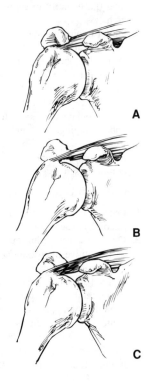

Fig. 12–1. Classification of rotator cuff tears. (A) Bursal surface tear, (B) articular surface tear, (C) intratendinous tear.

2. Complete Tears
   a. Total disruption of cuff fibers from bursal surface to articular surface
   b. Graded by size of tear or degree of retraction
      (1) Small = < 1 cm
      (2) Moderate = 1–3 cm
      (3) Large = 3–5 cm
      (4) Massive = > 5 cm
   c. Classifying full-thickness tears
      (1) Stage I: involves only supraspinatus tendon
      (2) Stage II: involves supraspinatus and infraspinatus tendons
      (3) Stage III: involves supraspinatus, infraspinatus, and subscapularis tendons
      (4) Stage IV: rotator cuff arthropathy

CLINICAL PRESENTATION

Impingement

1. Increasingly frequent and severe shoulder pain and stiffness
2. Symptoms usually associated with certain athletic activities
3. Elicit pain by overhead or across-body movement or throwing (impingement with or without deceleration pain)
4. Lifting in ''thumb down'' position (supraspinatus load) exacerbates symptoms
5. Night pain and morning stiffness
6. Point tenderness, especially at acromion's leading edge
7. Generalized shoulder pain or discomfort extending to deltoid insertion

Rotator Cuff Tears

1. Symptom pattern similar to impingement
2. Pain with activity and arm weakness
3. Crepitation, grinding, and popping
4. Severity of pain not predictive of tear size

PHYSICAL EXAMINATION

General Observations

1. Findings depend to some extent on degree of rotator cuff damage
2. Symptoms: mild tenderness, weakness, and pain on impingement test (Fig. 12–2) to profound atrophy and inability to actively raise arm
3. Tenderness localized to greater tuberosity and subacromial bursa
4. Biceps tendon inflamed and tender, and long head of biceps tendon may be ruptured

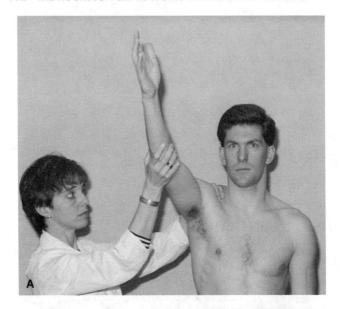

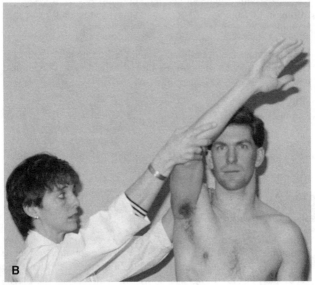

Fig. 12–2. Impingement sign.

5. Upper third of trapezius and deltoid insertion on humerus may be tender from referred pain and compensatory overuse
6. Painful active ROM throughout arc with painful passive ROM only at extremes
7. Differentiate shoulder stiffness from partial tears or chronic large complete tears from adhesive capsulitis

Strength Testing

1. Supraspinatus weakness in forward flexion and abduction very sensitive for rotator cuff tear if local anesthetic has ablated pain
2. Degree of weakness correlates well with tear size
3. Concomitant weakness in external rotation suggests involvement of infraspinatus
4. Some patients with massive tears cannot passively hold arm in external rotation
5. Measure deltoid, internal rotators, and biceps strength

Scapular Mechanics

1. Test for passive ROM of scapula and for scapular position under load (eg, wall pushup or abduction against resistance)
2. Look for asymmetric motion or tilt

AC Joint

1. Examine for tenderness and evidence of previous subluxation or spurring
2. Horizontal and overhead adduction cause pain

RADIOGRAPHIC EVALUATION

Plain Radiography

1. AP view in scapular plane in internal and external rotation: determines acromiohumeral distance (narrowed with some larger tears), acromial spurring and sclerosis, GH arthritis, and reactive changes at greater tuberosity
2. Supraspinatus outlet view: identifies acromial shape and distal clavicular spurring
3. Axillary view: helps identify os acromiale and GH joint narrowing

Arthrography

1. Radiographic dye leakage from GH joint into subacromial space indicates full-thickness tear, but tear size not always related to amount of dye leakage
2. Partial articular surface tears display thin stream of dye into tendon defect, but no extravasation into bursal space
3. Negative arthrogram does not exclude partial bursal surface or intra-tendinous tear

MRI

1. More definitive information about rotator cuff disorders, but expensive
2. Use when diagnosis cannot be made or confirmed by physical examination, plain radiography, or arthrography

TREATMENT

Criteria Based on Patient's Activity Level and Duration of Symptoms

1. Treat conservatively less active "nonoverhead" athletes and those with ≤ 3–6 mos of symptoms
2. Intervene early with active overhead athletes and those with ≥3 mos of symptoms

Conservative (Nonsurgical) Treatment

1. Appropriate for Stage I and early Stage II impingement lesions that have not disrupted rotator cuff
2. Smaller percentage of late Stage II and Stage III lesions respond to conservative treatment and may eventually require surgery
3. Most orthopedists recommend conservative treatment for all patients initially, except those with massive cuff avulsions and associated fractures needing early, more aggressive treatment
4. Inflammation control may require ↓ or elimination of exacerbating athletic activities, and NSAIDs
5. Modify overhead technique to ↓ rotator cuff compromise
6. Judicious local corticosteroid injections beneficial in treating rotator cuff lesions with tendinitis and partial tears
   a. Temporary pain relief from ↓ inflammation often allows for better participation in and ↑ benefit from exercise program to optimize motion and strength
   b. Do not inject steroids in patients with complete rotator cuff tears, especially if surgery eventually anticipated, as multiple injections (≥ 4) can weaken cuff tissue
7. Exercise program goals: to restore normal ROM and optimize rotator cuff, deltoid, and scapular muscle strength

RETURN TO ACTIVITY

1. Restrict until ROM restored, both rest- and activity-related pain eliminated, and provocative tests negative
2. Resume activities gradually; may need to modify work load or volume if symptoms recur
3. ↑ work load to return to full, unrestricted activities

4. Continue flexibility and strengthening exercises after return to sport to prevent recurrence

SURGICAL INTERVENTION

1. May be indicated for those who fail well-supervised rehab program
2. Options: arthroscopic, open, or combination, depending on bone and soft-tissue conditions anticipated or encountered during surgery
3. Surgery for rotator cuff tear relieves pain, but does not predictably improve function or strength
4. Results depend on repair quality, tissue quality, interval from injury to repair, size and extent of tear, associated neurologic injury, deltoid function, and disciplined postoperative therapy program
5. Results better when surgery earlier: muscle atrophy and contracture, arthritic changes, and progressive shoulder stiffness make surgery and rehab more difficult
6. For partial rotator cuff tears involving $< 50\%$ of tendon in patients with Type II or Type III acromion, arthroscopic or open surgery appropriate
7. In active, young patient with partial rotator cuff tear involving $> 50\%$ of tendon's thickness, open surgery preferred
8. Older, less active patients with large partial-thickness tears and minimal symptoms may only require arthroscopic surgery
9. Repair or reconstruct symptomatic complete rotator cuff tears
10. Even with surgery, massive rotator cuff tears often improve minimally in function because of continued rotator cuff deficiency; thus, limited-goals rehab program appropriate

13

Fractures and Dislocations about the Elbow

MEDIAL EPICONDYLE FRACTURES

Mechanism of Injury

1. Avulsion fracture can be from fall on extended upper extremity, but more often due to chronic valgus overload of elbow in adolescent throwing athlete (Fig. 13–1)
2. Commonly associated with elbow dislocation when due to fall
3. May reduce spontaneously
4. Usually occur in teenagers because medial epicondyle has not yet fused with distal humerus

Clinical Presentation

1. Pain localized to medial elbow or diffuse
2. Avulsion fractures → medial epicondyle tenderness and variable amounts of swelling
3. Neurologic compromise may occur because of ulnar nerve proximity to medial epicondyle
   a. Areas of paresthesia or small sensory deficits usually resolve on own
   b. Motor deficits, with or without sensory loss, require surgical intervention
4. ROM ↓ because of pain

Radiographic Evaluation

1. Obtain AP, lateral, and oblique radiographs
2. In skeletally immature athletes, may need comparative normal elbow views to diagnose minimally displaced fracture
3. Fracture usually involves only epicondyle, but small portion of metaphysis may be attached
   a. Epicondyle displaced distally (Fig. 13–2).
   b. Fracture usually occurs through apophysis, but may occur through epiphysis
4. Fragment may become entrapped in elbow joint

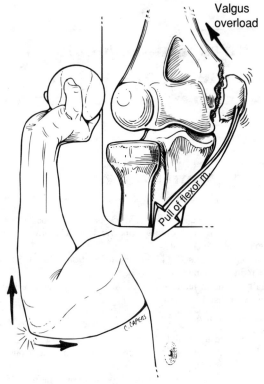

Fig. 13–1. Mechanism of injury of an avulsion fracture of the medial epicondyle. The pull of the forearm flexor group and the normal valgus elbow anatomy produce the fracture through the epicondylar apophysis.

    a. If at joint level, fragment not visible on radiographs
    b. Medial joint space widening indicates presence of fragment within joint
5. Arthrography confirms fragment entrapment
6. Gravity stress test radiograph determines valgus instability
    a. With patient supine and shoulder externally rotated, flex elbow 15–20°
    b. Significant medial opening with movement of fragment indicates medial instability

Treatment

1. Depends on amount of fracture displacement, valgus instability, whether fragment entrapped in joint, and presence of ulnar nerve injury

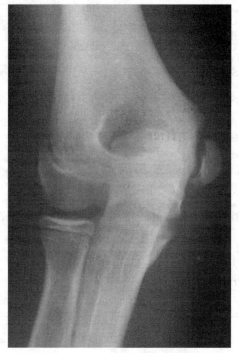

Fig. 13–2. Radiograph shows a medial epicondylar fracture.

2. Nondisplaced and Minimally Displaced (2–3 mm) Fractures
    a. Immobilize with posterior splint
    b. Start active assisted ROM exercises as early as 4–5 days after injury
    c. Discard splint once swelling and tenderness minimal
    d. Return to sports when full ROM and strength restored
3. Displaced Fractures without Valgus Instability, Entrapped Fragment, or Ulnar Nerve Injury
    a. Conservative treatment equal to or better than ORIF
    b. Treat as for nondisplaced or minimally displaced fracture, but wear posterior splint longer; still, keep use to minimum to attain full ROM
4. Surgical Intervention
    a. Remove entrapped fragments from joint and affix to medial condyle
    b. If ulnar nerve entrapped in joint or in fracture, re-attach medial epicondyle and perform ulnar nerve neurolysis with transposition

    c. If fracture results in valgus instability in athlete
      (1) Compare AP stress radiograph with normal AP radiograph
      (2) If fragment has moved, ORIF
      (3) Unrepaired medial instability disables athlete
    d. Postoperative Management
      (1) Start ROM as soon as pain permits (as early as 1 wk)
      (2) Remove splint in 3 wks
      (3) Start strengthening when full ROM attained
      (4) Return to throwing gradually within 6–8 wks

CORONOID FRACTURES

Mechanism of Injury

1. Violent brachialis muscle contraction
2. Occurs with forced elbow extension while brachialis contracts to prevent extension

Classification: Based on percentage of coronoid involved

1. Type I = < 25%
2. Type II = 25–50%
3. Type III = > 50%

Clinical Presentation

1. Anterior elbow swelling and tenderness with pain on extension
2. Often associated with elbow dislocation, radial head fracture, and medial ligament disruption
   Physical Examination: Perform complete neurovascular and stability examination for elbow dislocation.

Radiographic Evaluation

1. Obtain AP, lateral, and oblique views
2. If fracture not revealed, obtain radiocapitellar view

Treatment

1. Type I fractures: nonsurgical
   a. Immobilize elbow for 3–4 days, then start ROM exercises
   b. Therapy progression and return to sports dictated by symptoms
   c. No protection needed for sports
2. Type II or III fractures with associated elbow dislocation or multiple fractures: ORIF
3. Large coronoid fractures: anatomic reduction to prevent elbow instability

OLECRANON FRACTURES

Mechanism of Injury

1. Olecranon process especially vulnerable to direct trauma because of subcutaneous location

2. Three mechanisms of injury
   a. Direct trauma (eg, fall on elbow point)
   b. Indirect trauma (eg, fall on outstretched hand with elbow flexed, with strong triceps contraction)
   c. Combination of direct and indirect trauma

Classification

1. Nondisplaced
   a. $<$ 2 mm displacement
   b. No ↑ separation with 90° flexion
   c. Able to extend elbow actively against gravity
2. Displaced

Clinical Presentation

1. Effusion causes swelling and olecranon pain
2. Most important sign: inability to extend elbow actively against gravity indicates disruption of triceps mechanism

Radiographic Evaluation

1. True lateral view needed to detect fracture
2. AP view delineates fracture line in sagittal plane

Treatment

1. Nondisplaced fractures
   a. Immobilize in long-arm cast with elbow flexed 45–90°
   b. Start movement after 3 wks, but avoid flexion past 90° until bone healing complete (6–8 wks)
2. Displaced fractures: ORIF or primary excision

RADIAL HEAD FRACTURES

Mechanism of Injury

1. Direct blow or fall on outstretched hand
2. During elbow dislocation

Classification (Fig. 13–3)

1. Type I: marginal fracture without displacement
2. Type II: marginal fracture with displacement
3. Type III: comminuted fracture of entire head
4. Type IV: any radial head fracture with elbow dislocation

Clinical Presentation

1. Diffuse swelling from joint hemarthrosis
2. Radial head tenderness and pain on palpation
3. ↓ ROM from pain, swelling, or loose bodies

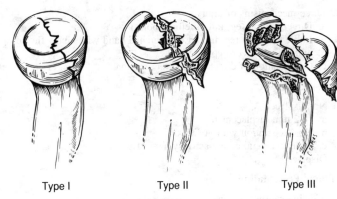

Type I   Type II   Type III

Fig. 13–3. Classification of radial head fractures. Type I, marginal fracture without displacement; Type II, marginal fracture with displacement; Type III, comminuted entire head fracture.

Physical Examination

1. Aspirate hemarthrosis and inject local anesthetic
2. If anesthesia does not allow full ROM, suspect loose body
3. For Type II, III, or IV fractures, examine wrist for possible radioulnar dissociation, which signifies ↑ degree of injury

Radiographic Evaluation

1. Obtain AP and lateral views
2. If no fracture seen, but posterior fat pad sign present, obtain radiocapitellar view
3. If wrist pain, obtain wrist series
4. CT can further delineate fracture

Treatment

1. Type I
   a. Symptomatic treatment and early ROM
   b. Aspirate hemarthrosis and inject local anesthetic
   c. Place arm in sling for 2–3 days
   d. Start flexion and extension first, then pronation and supination
   e. Attain full ROM early
   f. Allow full return to activity when painless ROM is full (usually within 2–3 mos).
   g. No protective equipment required
2. Type II: treatment depends on fracture pattern
   a. Type II with ≤ 2 mm or less displacement: treat closed, as for Type I
   b. Type II with no comminution, but > 2 mm displacement: ORIF

3. Type III: ORIF
4. If fracture fragment < 25–30% of radial head and mechanical block present, excise fragment
5. If no mechanical block, splint forearm in full supination for 2–3 wks to allow interosseous membrane to heal
6. In Types I and II and some Type III fractures, can excise fragment arthroscopically; do not perform arthroscopy if other related injuries (eg, elbow dislocation or medial instability) present

Functional Anatomy

Acute elbow instability is more common in sports that impose upper extremity stress. If active and passive elbow constraints are compromised, instability can occur. Valgus instability (from acute or chronic process) is caused wholly or partially by compromise of medial collateral ligament complex (MCL). The essential functional element of this complex: anterior oblique component.

ACUTE DISLOCATION

Mechanism of Injury

1. Acute elbow instability (ie, dislocation or fracture-dislocation) usually from fall on outstretched arm or direct trauma
2. Valgus, supination, and hyperextension stresses to elbow result in posteromedial or posterolateral dislocation of ulna relative to distal humerus
3. Anterior dislocation (rare) usually associated with proximal olecranon fracture
4. Even rarer: divergent dislocation 2° to compromise of annular ligament and interosseous membrane

Clinical Presentation

1. Swollen, disfigured extremity
2. Neurovascular deficits in 2–4%, most often 2° to ulnar nerve lesion
3. Associated injuries: shoulder, elbow, or wrist fractures
4. Open injuries uncommon

Radiographic Evaluation

1. Defines dislocation type and any associated fractures
2. Important to recognize associated injuries to prevent longterm dysfunction
3. If dislocation spontaneously reduces, only soft tissue swelling may be seen; perform valgus gravity stress testing (Fig. 13–4); medial joint widening > 1–2 mm or valgus angulation > 7° over contralateral side indicates probable dislocation

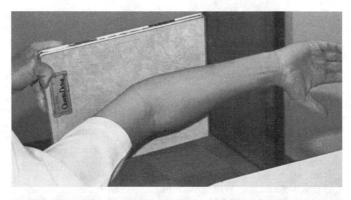

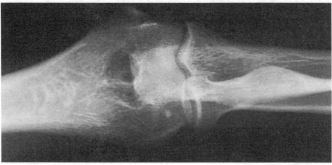

Fig. 13–4. Gravity stress testing can be used to detect spontaneous dislocation of the elbow.

Treatment

1. Early reduction and treatment of any associated injuries
   a. Primary open reduction not indicated for simple dislocation with congruous reduction
   b. Open management may be needed if dislocation > 3 wks old; closed reduction usually impossible by then
2. Perform reduction in ER with IV sedation or in OR when fractures or neurovascular injuries are associated or when general anesthesia required
3. Reduction method similar in either case
   a. Apply longitudinal traction to forearm and wrist while holding elbow slightly flexed
   b. Reduce posterolateral or posteromedial dislocations by manual translation

c. Apply gentle traction to unlock coronoid from olecranon fossa; may require posterior translation of proximal forearm relative to distal humerus by assistant

d. Note reduction as sigmoid notch snaps onto trochlea

4. Postreduction radiographs and physical examination document congruous reduction

5. Then put extremity through ROM to test joint stability
   a. Stable joint
      (1) Splint elbow for few days for pain control
      (2) Then start early active ROM exercises; early mobilization important to prevent flexion contractures
   b. Unstable joint
      (1) Use extension block initially
      (2) Gradually ↓ use of block over 2–3 wks

6. Concomitant lateral column fractures require either internal fixation or prosthetic replacement

7. Treat concomitant wrist fractures aggressively to allow early elbow ROM and ↓ period of immobilization

8. Postreduction management of simple dislocations
   a. Avoid early passive ROM exercises that exacerbate tissue trauma and may result in heterotopic ossification
   b. Start active ROM exercises within 1st wk as swelling ↓
   c. Range should approach 80–100° arc within 2 wks
   d. Place no limit on flexion
   e. Limit extension at first only if instability noted
   f. Institute active assisted program 2 wks after initiation of ROM if restoration of motion slower than expected
   g. If flexion contracture present at 4–6 wks, extension orthosis can help restore full extension
   h. Start strengthening program at 6–8 wks, but avoid loading elbow until strength restored and ROM within 30° of preinjury capability (usually 2–3 months)
   i. Generally, athletes return to play within 3–6 months

CHRONIC POSTEROLATERAL ROTATORY INSTABILITY (MOST COMMON FORM OF CHRONIC INSTABILITY)

Mechanism of Injury: acute frank or near elbow dislocation
Clinical Presentation: apprehension and posterolateral elbow pain when elbow bears valgus axial load and forearm is supinated

Physical Examination

1. Posterolateral pivot shift test (Fig. 13–5): best performed with general anesthesia because of patient apprehension

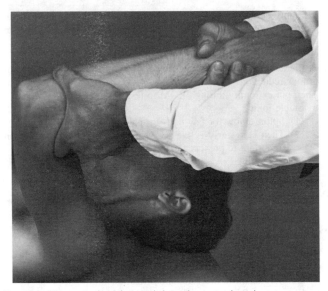

Fig. 13–5. The posterolateral pivot shift test for posterolateral rotatory instability.

2. Hyperflex shoulder to lock shoulder girdle
3. Apply valgus, supination, and axial compression loads to elbow
4. With elbow extended, subluxation or dislocation of radius and proximal ulna (noted by radial head prominence and sulcus sign) evident
5. Then flex elbow and note palpable or audible click as radial head reduces on capitellum

   Radiographic Evaluation: usually negative, except for occasional evidence of avulsion fractures of lateral epicondyle

Treatment

1. If detected very early after injury, apply extension block orthosis with forearm pronated; however, rarely is lesion detected early enough to validate this treatment method
2. If confirmed under general anesthesia, surgical reconstruction required; most patients have successful outcome; nonsurgical management not effective
3. Postoperative management
   a. Place extremity in long-arm cast with elbow in 90° flexion and forearm fully pronated
   b. Wear cast for 4 wks, then change to hinged cast with extension block of 30° for 6 wks

   c. Remove extension block if no evidence of ligamentous laxity
   d. Younger patients or those with generalized laxity may need extension block splinting for as long as 6 mos
   e. Use splint for minimum of 3 mos postoperatively, then allow ROM exercises in forearm rotation
   f. No loaded activities or extension past neutral for at least 6 mos postoperatively

CHRONIC MEDIAL INSTABILITY

Mechanism of Injury: common in athletes whose sports place repetitive valgus stress on elbow (eg, baseball pitchers)

Clinical Presentation

1. Medial elbow pain after repeated throwing
2. Acute episode with sharp pain may occur, but chronic progressive course more typical
3. Most severe pain in cocking and acceleration phases of throwing
4. Lateral elbow pain, especially in younger athletes: compromise of medial stabilizers results in overload of lateral stabilizer
5. Ulnar neuropathy paresthesias in ulnar distribution of hand
6. Forced palmar flexion of wrist and forearm rotation may result in concomitant medial epicondylitis

Physical Examination

1. Test MCL by applying valgus stress to elbow in 25° flexion (Fig. 13–6)
   a. Hold patient's hand and wrist in examiner's axilla, against trunk with upper arm
   b. Cup hands at elbow level, with 1 thumb on inferior margin of medial epicondyle along MCL
   c. With other hand, apply valgus stress to elbow
   d. Pain with this maneuver (with or without gross laxity) confirms MCL dysfunction
   e. Perform test with forearm pronated to prevent false-positive finding representing medial epicondylitis (not uncommon for conditions to coexist)
2. Perform Tinel's nerve percussion test and elbow flexion test to assess ulnar neuropathy at elbow
3. Assess 2-point discrimination and hand intrinsic muscle strength

Radiographic Evaluation

1. Assesses articular dysfunction
2. Gravity stress testing or applied loads verify gross ligamentous laxity

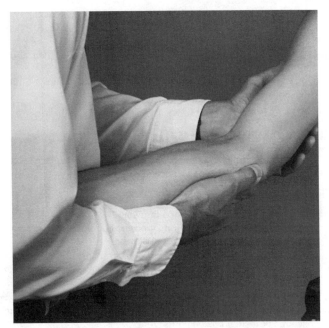

Fig. 13–6. The medial collateral ligament is tested by placing valgus stress on the elbow with the joint in 25° of flexion, to unlock the olecranon from its fossa.

Treatment

1. In most cases, attempt nonsurgical treatment initially
2. Conservative management likely to be successful in mild cases and those with brief history of symptoms
3. Conservative management
   a. Rest, avoid valgus and pronation stress, and NSAIDs
   b. Start stretching program for flexor-pronator mass as pain subsides
   c. Perform pronation and wrist palmar flexion strengthening exercises incrementally
   d. Gradually resume throwing activity after several wks rest
   e. If pain does not recur, return to full activity
   f. If pain recurs, slow down rehab
   g. Counterforce bracing for medial epicondylitis may help
4. Preventive measures
   a. Preactivity stretching
   b. Strengthening program to maximize active stabilizers of elbow

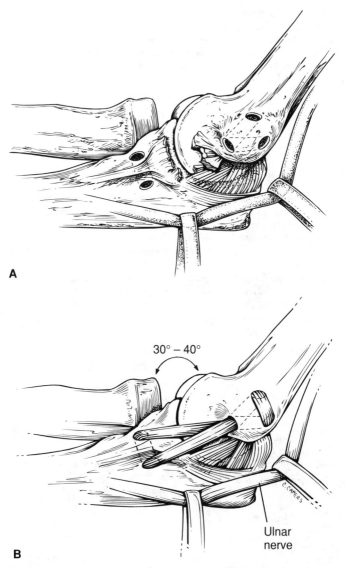

Fig. 13–7. The medial collateral ligament is reconstructed with palmaris longus tendon graft through drill holes. The graft is sutured with the elbow in 30° to 40° of flexion in a figure-of-eight pattern, doubling the graft across the joint.

   c. Ice after activity
   d. Modify exacerbating activities
5. Avoid corticosteroid injections for medial epicondylitis, as they may predispose to acute rupture of flexor-pronator mass; corticosteroid injection into MCL proper contraindicated
6. Surgical intervention
   a. If extended conservative management fails to restore elbow to preinjury status, surgical reconstruction of MCL indicated (Fig. 13–7)
   b. Surgical decompression of ulnar nerve may also be necessary
7. Postoperative management
   a. Immobilize for 2 wks
   b. Start digital active ROM program immediately postop
   c. Start active elbow ROM at 2 wks
   d. Start digital- and forearm-strengthening program at 4–6 wks
   e. Start elbow strengthening at 8 wks after surgery, avoiding valgus stress (no active internal or passive external rotation of shoulder)
8. Return to activity
   a. Gradually ↑ distance, frequency, duration, and velocity of pitching postop
   b. Resume competitive pitching 1 yr postop at earliest if progress optimal; often takes up to 18 mos to regain preinjury level
   c. Even with carefully supervised rehab, only $\frac{2}{3}$ of high-demand athletes regain preinjury levels

SUMMARY

1. Acute elbow instability 2° to simple dislocation
   a. Very good prognosis for return to preinjury level
   b. Anticipate recovery within 6 mos
2. Instability due to fracture-dislocation
   a. Less favorable prognosis depending on nature of fracture
   b. Chronic instability usually requires surgical reconstruction and longer recovery
3. Elbow instability often career-altering or career-ending injury, even when managed properly

Overuse Injuries of the Elbow in the Throwing Athlete

THROWING INJURIES OF THE MEDIAL ELBOW
Flexor-Pronator Muscle Strains

1. Mechanism of Injury
   a. Repeated valgus stress leads to inflammation or even microscopic tearing of flexor muscles at attachment to medial humeral epicondyle
   b. Cocking and acceleration phases generate medial tension and lateral compression forces at elbow (Fig. 14–1)
   c. Repetitive trauma to chronically fatigued muscle can → microscopic tearing and pain
   d. Complete ruptures of flexor musculature rare
2. Clinical Presentation
   a. Pain, tenderness, and swelling over medial elbow, usually after workout or throwing
   b. Inability to fully extend elbow
   c. Active resisted wrist flexion or forearm pronation produces medial elbow pain
3. Treatment
   a. Treat short-duration symptoms that occur only after throwing with ice, NSAIDs, and rest from exacerbating activities
   b. Apply heat after approximately 36 hrs
   c. Phonophoresis and galvanic stimulation may help
   d. Fully extend elbow and extend and supinate wrist to stretch wrist flexors and pronators
   e. Corticosteroid injections rarely, if ever, indicated
   f. In more resistant cases, in which injury due to force overload from faulty mechanics and improper throwing technique, modify throwing motion

MEDIAL HUMERAL EPICONDYLITIS (MEDIAL OR REVERSE TENNIS ELBOW)

1. Mechanism of injury: variant of flexor-pronator strain
2. Clinical presentation

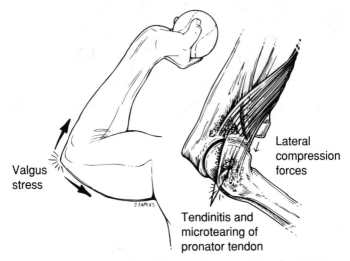

Fig. 14–1. During the act of throwing, medial tension and lateral compression forces are applied to the elbow. These forces can lead to microscopic tearing and pain.

   a. More proximal and discretely localized pain, predominantly over tip of medial humeral epicondyle
   b. Occasionally, more distal tenderness for about 2.5 cm along pronator teres and flexor carpi radialis insertion
   c. Resisted testing of flexor-pronator group may or may not cause medial elbow pain
3. Treatment
   a. Mild cases: ice, NSAIDs, stretching and strengthening, rest from painful activities, and avoid further force overload
   b. More serious cases with greater pathologic changes: biologic healing must occur to relieve pain, and rehab may stimulate healing as long as overload force avoided
   c. Inject mixture of local anesthetic and corticosteroid into area of maximum tenderness over medial humeral epicondyle if other treatment modalities fail
      (1) Avoid ulnar nerve, located posterior to epicondyle
      (2) Give no more than 3 injections at 1-month intervals, and emphasize rest, stretching, and strengthening
   d. Surgical intervention rarely necessary

MEDIAL COLLATERAL LIGAMENT (MCL) INJURIES

1. Mechanism of injury: seen most often in baseball pitchers, javelin throwers, and football quarterbacks

2. Clinical Presentation
   a. Sprain
      (1) Medial elbow pain directly over anterior band of MCL
      (2) No history of significant trauma
   b. Acute rupture
      (1) History: traumatic valgus thrust applied to medial elbow, resulting in audible pop
      (2) Unable to continue throwing because of acute medial elbow pain
      (3) Possible associated ulnar nerve symptoms: paresthesia in ring and little fingers or weakness of hand
      (4) Tenderness and swelling along medial elbow at MCL
      (5) Ecchymosis usually, but may be delayed up to 72 hrs
      (6) Valgus stress of elbow produces medial pain
3. Radiographic Evaluation of Acute Rupture
   a. Gravity stress test can demonstrate medial elbow opening
   b. CT arthrogram and MRI help document injury
4. Treatment
   a. Sprain
      (1) Ice, NSAIDs, and complete rest from throwing for 2–3 wks
      (2) When pain resolves, gradual return to throwing
   b. Acute rupture: immediate surgical exploration and ligament repair or reconstruction
   c. Chronic insufficiency
      (1) Elbow and wrist endurance strengthening (both concentric and eccentric), stretching, NSAIDs, and occasional rest from normal activities
      (2) Evaluate and correct any improper pitching and throwing mechanics and techniques
      (3) If conservative measures fail and throwing-related pain or instability continues, consider surgical reconstruction of MCL for throwing athletes who want to remain active; after surgery, may need 8–12 mos of rehab
      (4) Some believe surgery should only be salvage procedure for limited future playing; returning player with chronic elbow arthritis to high levels of throwing after reconstruction may → recurrent symptoms and further degenerative changes

THROWING INJURIES OF THE LATERAL ELBOW

Lateral Humeral Epicondylitis (Tendinosis or tennis elbow)

1. Mechanism of Injury
   a. Tensile stresses over the lateral epicondyle produce inflammation or partial tearing of extensor musculature
   b. These stresses occur during extreme forearm pronation and wrist flexion in release and deceleration phases

    c. Lateral elbow inflammation also caused by overuse in batting practice or associated with weight training injuries

    d. More degenerative process than acute inflammatory process or one associated with single injury

2. Clinical Presentation

    a. History of weak grip and gradual onset of pain just distal to lateral humeral epicondyle

    b. Pain from activities of daily living that require wrist extension

    c. Reproduce symptoms by

        (1) Extending wrist against resistance with elbow slightly flexed

        (2) Passive stretching of extensor carpi radialis brevis by full elbow extension and wrist flexion

    d. Tenderness along muscle belly of extensor carpi radialis brevis

    e. Swelling and ecchymosis not prominent

3. Radiographic Evaluation: usually normal, although lateral soft-tissue calcifications may be seen

4. Treatment

    a. Ice, NSAIDs, rest from painful activities, and wrist extensor stretching and endurance strengthening

    b. Counterforce bracing of extensor carpi radialis brevis, phonophoresis, and galvanic stimulation

    c. Corticosteroid injections (3 over 3–6 mos) just under aponeurosis, not in musculotendinous area, as last resort

    d. If pain continues after 6 months' conservative treatment, surgery may be indicated

OSTEOCHONDRITIS DISSECANS OF THE CAPITELLUM

1. Mechanism of Injury

    a. Articular cartilage and underlying subchondral bone of capitellum undergo inflammation, swelling, fragmentation, occasional loose body formation, and secondary degenerative changes throughout elbow

    b. Changes may be caused by repetitive compression loads producing fragmentation or vascular disruption

2. Classification

    a. Stage I

        (1) Children up to 13 yrs

        (2) Lesion seldom fragments

        (3) Minimal symptoms

    b. Stage II

        (1) Age 13 to adult

        (2) History of prolonged competition and repetitive throwing activities

        (3) Pronounced symptoms

    c. Stage III

    (1) Adults
    (2) Poorest prognosis
    (3) Symptoms present for yrs
    (4) Capitellar fragments, loose bodies, joint incongruity, and secondary degenerative changes

3. Clinical Presentation
  a. Insidious onset and progression of symptoms
  b. Localized pain, ↓ ROM (particularly extension) , swelling, catching, and occasional locking and crepitus, usually associated with attempts at full extension or forearm supination

4. Radiographic Evaluation
  a. Demonstrates capitellar fragmentation and associated loose bodies
  b. In younger patients, MRI can demonstrate articular cartilage involvement and may reveal stable or unstable osteochondral fragments

5. Treatment
  a. Stage I: Restrict throwing if there is pain and locking; prolonged elbow rest (6–12 mos) may be necessary
  b. Stage II: ↓ activity level; if catching, pain, and loose body sensation present, consider arthroscopic debridement and loose body removal
  c. Stage III: ↓ activity level, NSAIDs, and perhaps arthroscopic debridement and loose body removal

POSTERIOR ELBOW

Triceps Tendinitis: treat with ice, NSAIDs, rest, stretching, and strengthening

Minor Triceps Avulsion Fractures: May present as persistent posterior elbow pain when joint is fully extended

VALGUS EXTENSION OVERLOAD SYNDROME

Mechanism of Injury

1. Affects posterior and posteromedial elbow
2. Valgus and extension stresses to elbow produce olecranon impingement, resulting in pain
  a. Pain occurs during release and deceleration phases
  b. As elbow extends, medial olecranon impinges against posteromedial olecranon fossa (Fig. 14–2)
  c. Valgus laxity from UCL stretching alters throwing mechanics and can worsen syndrome

Clinical Presentation

1. Baseball pitchers
  a. History of elbow pain after pitching

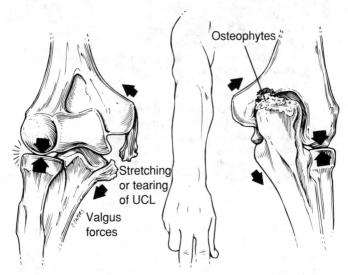

Fig. 14–2. Valgus extension overload usually occurs in the release and deceleration phases of throwing. The medial aspect of the olecranon impinges against the posteromedial aspect of the olecranon fossa as the elbow is brought into extension. Stretching or tearing of the ulnar collateral ligament (UCL) leads to valgus laxity and can worsen the problem.

   b. Loss of control and fatigue after 2–3 innings
   c. Most pain occurs as pitcher attempts to ''whip'' arm to gain maximum speed
2. Pain over posterior elbow with forced extension and valgus loading
3. Occasionally, posterior olecranon pain and swelling
4. More advanced cases: locking and catching

Radiographic Evaluation

1. Obtain AP, lateral, and oblique views
2. Obtain radiographic ''olecranon'' or axial view to demonstrate osteophytes

Treatment

1. Conservative: ice, NSAIDs, relative rest from throwing, stretching, and other modalities
2. If symptoms persist and athlete wants to continue throwing, consider surgical intervention

ANTERIOR ELBOW

Anterior Capsular Strain or Mild Insertional Biceps Strain

1. Caused by elbow hyperextension
2. Treat with ice, NSAIDs, rest, and gentle stretching; avoid hyperextension whenever possible

Chronic Flexion Contractures of the Elbow

1. Not incompatible with normal functioning and throwing
2. Surgery generally unsuccessful and not usually indicated

LITTLE LEAGUER'S ELBOW

Mechanism of Injury

1. Multiple pathologic processes in adolescent thrower's elbow caused by medial tension–lateral compression forces placed on elbow during throwing

Clinical Presentation

1. History of nonspecific pain during or after throwing and occasional loss of control
2. Prolonged joint stiffness and ↓ ROM
3. Diffuse tenderness, occasional swelling, and at times ↑ elbow valgus

Radiographic Evaluation

1. May reveal medial humeral epicondyle overgrowth and fragmentation, osteochondritis dissecans of capitellum, generalized trabecular and cortical thickening of bony structures of elbow, and loose bodies
2. Both symptomatic and asymptomatic patients may have abnormal radiographs

Treatment

1. If radiographs normal, treat symptoms with rest, ice, and stretching; no return to pitching until all symptoms subside
2. If radiographs show abnormalities associated with throwing, stop throwing; surgery may be indicated for removal of loose bodies or debridement of osteochondritis dissecans

THROWING NEUROPATHIES OF THE ELBOW AND FOREARM

Ulnar Nerve

1. Mechanism of Injury
   a. Most often thrower develops ulnar nerve symptoms from mechan-

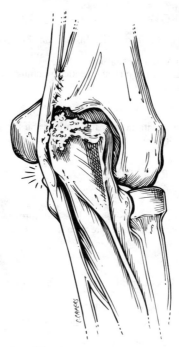

Fig. 14–3. Compression of the ulnar nerve.

ical compromise of nerve medially from traction friction or compression

(1) ↓ nerve movement allows compression or tethering during throwing (Fig. 14–3)

(2) Repeated nerve trauma produces inflammation, adhesions, and further restriction of normal movement

(3) Fibrosis and vascular compromise can result

b. Other Causes

(1) Direct nerve trauma

(2) Repetitive traction injury 2° to cubitus valgus alignment or associated with UCL laxity

(3) Nerve hypermobility with recurrent subluxation or dislocation

(4) Medial soft tissue calcification or ossification

(5) Acute UCL tear

(6) Epicondylar fracture or separation

2. Clinical Presentation

a. Posteromedial elbow pain and heavy feeling of hand

    b. Tingling or paresthesia over ulnar distribution to ring and little fingers and (+) Tinel's sign

    c. Sensory deficits in ulnar half of ring and little fingers, palmar hypothenar area, and dorsal ulnar aspect of hand

    d. No motor weakness initially

    e. Swelling and tenderness in ulnar groove

3. Treatment

    a. Rest for 2–3 wks, splinting, and NSAIDs; return to throwing when asymptomatic

    b. Anterior transposition of ulnar nerve indicated

       (1) For patients who fail conservative treatment, have prolonged symptoms, and wish to continue throwing

       (2) If electromyographic evidence of neuropathy or clinical evidence of motor weakness

       (3) At time of UCL repair or reconstruction

MEDIAN NERVE

1. Mechanism of Injury: direct trauma or repetitive stress
2. Clinical Presentation

    a. As pronator teres syndrome if compressed in proximal forearm

    b. As anterior interosseous syndrome if compressed more distally in forearm

3. Treatment

    a. Conservative: stretching, rest, NSAIDs, and correction of throwing technique and equipment (eg, racquet size and grip)

    b. If symptoms prolonged and disabling, consider surgical exploration and release of any structures impinging on nerve

RADIAL NERVE

1. Mechanism of Injury: direct trauma or muscular exertion during throwing
2. Treatment

    a. Stretching, rest, and NSAIDs

    b. Surgery, reserved for more resistant cases, to explore and release any impinging structures

Fractures and Dislocations of the Wrist, Hand, and Fingers

CARPAL INJURY

General Principles

1. Mechanism of Injury: Loading of wrist in extreme hyperextension
2. Classification (perilunate pattern of wrist injury)
   a. Stage 1: Scapholunate dissociation
   b. Stage 2: Includes capitate-lunate dislocation
   c. Stage 3: Includes triquetral dislocation
   d. Stage 4: Complete lunate dislocation
3. Two-Part Classification System
   a. Carpal Instability Dissociative (CID): complete ligamentous disruptions with proximal carpal row instability, including scapholunate and lunotriquetral dissociation
   b. Carpal Instability Nondissociative (CIND): collapse despite continued integrity of intrinsic ligaments; results from malunion and malalignment of distal radial fracture and from disruption or attenuation of extrinsic palmar ligaments

Scapholunate Instability

1. Mechanism of Injury
   a. Fall onto outstretched wrist → hyperextension, ulnar deviation, and supination
   b. Results in loss of support of proximal scaphoid pole through rupture of its ligamentous restraints
2. Clinical Presentation
   a. Pain, swelling, and tenderness over dorsoradial wrist
   b. (+) Watson's test (Fig. 15–1)
      (1) Ulnarly deviate wrist, then radially deviate while maintaining pressure on distal scaphoid pole
      (2) Unstable scaphoid subluxates dorsally and is painful
3. Radiographic Evaluation
   a. Classic sign: > 2 mm gap between scaphoid and lunate ("Terry Thomas" sign)

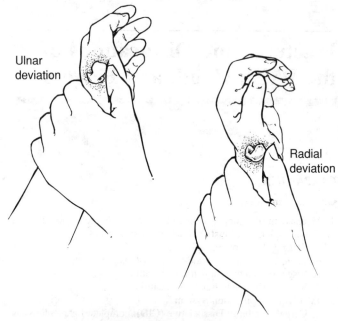

Fig. 15–1. In Watson's test for scaphoid instability, the examiner brings the patient's wrist into ulnar deviation. Then the patient's wrist is radially deviated while the examiner maintains pressure on the distal pole of the scaphoid. An unstable scaphoid will subluxate dorsally and be painful.

    b. End-on view of distal pole of perpendicular scaphoid seen as cortical "ring" sign

    c. Lateral view may reveal dorsiflexion instability pattern with scaphoid in vertical position and corresponding scapholunate angle > 65–70°

4. Treatment

    a. Treat acute and chronic dissociations surgically

    b. Return to competition within 4–8 wks

    c. Protect wrist with orthosis (eg, silicone cast) for 4–6 mos

Medial Carpal Instabilities

1. Triquetrohamate Instability

    a. Mechanism of injury: wrist dorsiflexion → disruption of arcuate ligament's capitotriquetral arm

    b. Clinical presentation: audible, palpable, and often painful "clunk" as wrist is moved from radial to ulnar deviation; point tenderness over triquetrohamate interspace

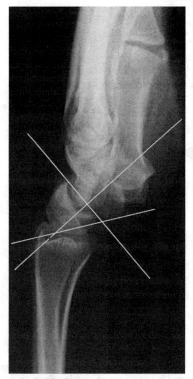

Fig. 15–2. Radiograph showing volarflexion instability pattern.

    c. Radiographic evaluation: volarflexion (Fig. 15–2) or dorsiflexion instability pattern, depending on wrist position

2. Triquetrolunate Instability

    a. Mechanism of injury: wrist dorsiflexion

    b. Clinical presentation: point tenderness over triquetrolunate joint; (+) ballottement test (stabilize lunate while attempting to displace triquetrum dorsally) (Fig. 15–3)

    c. Radiographic evaluation

        (1) Acute radiographs: normal

        (2) Chronic injury: volarflexion instability pattern

        (3) Arthrography: tear of lunotriquetral interosseous ligament

3. Treatment

    a. Treat most acute injuries conservatively: immobilize in above-elbow cast and NSAIDs

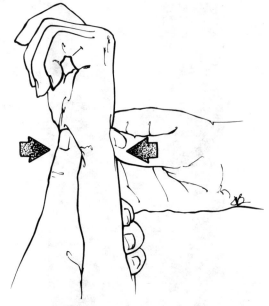

Fig. 15–3. With the ballottement test, the examiner stabilizes the lunate while attempting to displace the triquetrum dorsally.

    b. Treat well-defined acute ligamentous tear with percutaneous pinning followed by cast immobilization for 6–8 wks

    c. In chronic cases, arthrodesis recommended, but throwing athletes will lose wrist motion

    d. Return to competition in 6–12 wks

    e. Protect wrist with removable orthosis for 6 mos after injury

FRACTURES OF THE CARPAL BONES

Scaphoid Fractures

1. Mechanism of injury: wrist must be dorsiflexed at least 95°, with primary force to radial palm

2. Clinical presentation: wrist pain and tenderness over dorsal snuffbox or directly over scaphoid

3. Radiographic evaluation

    a. Posteroanterior and posterior oblique views with wrist in ulnar deviation

    b. If no fracture seen but symptoms persist, repeat radiographs at 1 and 3 wks

4. Treatment
    a. Most acute, nondisplaced fractures will heal if properly immobilized for appropriate length of time
    b. Stable fracture (ie, minimal displacement and angulation)
        (1) Immobilize with short arm-thumb spica cast (change every 4 wks for good fit) for 12–16 wks
        (2) Immobilize and protect wrist (eg, with rigid, removable splint) from impact loading for additional 3 mos
        (3) Return to competition based on fracture pattern, type of sport, level and degree of competition, and awareness of added risk
    c. Unstable fracture (ie, displacement > 1 mm or angulation with abnormal carpal alignment)
        (1) Depends on degree of instability and late presentation
        (2) Some can be treated with closed reduction, followed by long arm-thumb spica cast for 6 wks and conversion to short arm-thumb spica cast for 6 wks
        (3) Others require ORIF with immobilization for at least 8–12 wks
        (4) After initial immobilization and healing, protect wrist from impact loading with rigid, removable splint for 3 mos

Hamate Fractures

1. Mechanism of injury: direct trauma to hypothenar region of hand
2. Clinical presentation
    a. Persistent pain, ulnar wrist and proximal palm
    b. Tenderness over end of hamate hook in hypothenar eminence
    c. Forceful grip activities most affected
3. Radiographic evaluation
    a. Routine radiographs: no fracture
    b. Obtain carpal tunnel view (Fig. 15–4) and supination oblique wrist view
4. Treatment

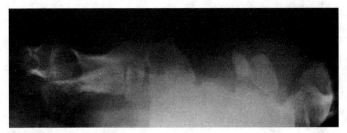

Fig. 15–4. Carpal tunnel view showing a hook of hamate fracture.

  a. Excise bony process
  b. Return to activity when pain and tenderness ↓ (6–8 wks)

Capitate Fractures

1. Mechanism of injury: extreme flexion or extension forces to wrist, combined with axial loading
2. Clinical presentation: swelling, point tenderness, pain, and loss of motion
3. Radiographic evaluation
  a. Plain radiographs usually show fracture
  b. Occasionally, oblique views used to define fracture plane
4. Treatment
  a. Immobilize nondisplaced fractures for 6 wks
  b. Displaced fractures usually require ORIF

Lunate Fractures

1. Mechanism of injury: repetitive trauma resulting in compression fracture
2. Radiographic evaluation: difficult to detect by plain films and may require bone scan, CT, or MRI
3. Treatment: immobilize for 8 wks

Pisiform Fractures

1. Mechanism of injury: direct trauma to hypothenar eminence
2. Treatment: immobilize with short-arm cast for 4–6 wks

Trapezium Fractures

1. Mechanism of injury: trapezial body compressed with radial deviation between 1st MCP and radial styloid
2. Treatment
  a. Immobilize nondisplaced fractures with cast for 6 wks
  b. Closed reduction and pinning or ORIF for displaced fractures

Triquetral Fractures

1. Usually chip or avulsion fractures
2. Treatment
  a. Splint for 4–6 wks
  b. Treat persistently painful, malunited chip fracture by excising fragment

INJURY TO THE DISTAL PHALANX

1. Mechanism of Injury: crushed fingertip with resultant fracture of distal phalanx (usually nondisplaced with no intra-articular involvement)
2. Treatment

a. Compressive dressing and finger splint protect and relieve pain
b. Drain subungual hematoma by piercing nail with heated paper clip to alleviate pressure and pain
c. If fracture displaced, replace nail matrix and repair anatomically

INJURIES TO THE DISTAL INTERPHALANGEAL (DIP) JOINT

Mallet Finger

1. Mechanism of Injury
   a. Avulsion of extensor tendon when DIP joint forcibly hyperflexed (Fig. 15-5), with or without concomitant avulsion of bone fragment from its insertion on distal phalanx
   b. Occurs when finger tip struck by ball
2. Clinical Presentation
   a. Characteristically dropped finger and inability to fully extend distal phalanx (full passive extension, however, usually possible)
   b. Local swelling and tenderness over dorsal DIP joint
3. Radiographic Evaluation: rule out fracture or joint subluxation if avulsion fracture present
4. Treatment
   a. If extensor tendon avulsed, splint finger dorsally with DIP joint in full extension or hyperextension and PIP joint in 60° flexion for 6 wks; continue splint for 2–3 more wks if DIP joint cannot actively extend
   b. Concomitant avulsion of large bone fragment or joint subluxation requires ORIF

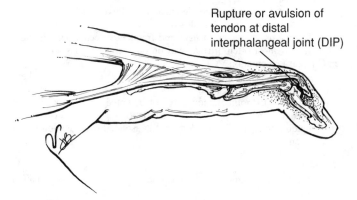

Rupture or avulsion of tendon at distal interphalangeal joint (DIP)

Fig. 15–5. Mallet finger describes an avulsion of the extensor tendon that occurs when the DIP joint is forcibly hyperflexed.

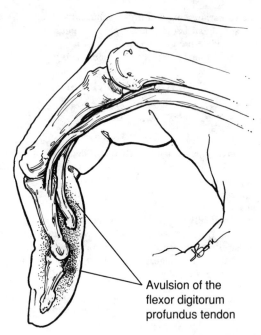

Avulsion of the
flexor digitorum
profundus tendon

Fig. 15–6. Avulsion of the flexor digitorum profundus tendon of the DIP joint.

Avulsion of the Flexor Digitorum Profundus Tendon

1. Mechanism of Injury
   a. Hyperextension force applied to actively flexed DIP joint ruptures tendon at insertion (Fig. 15–6)
   b. Known as ''sweater'' finger and frequently seen when athlete's finger (most often 3rd) catches on opposing player's jersey
2. Clinical Presentation
   a. Tender mass may be palpable in palm or proximal finger where avulsed tendon retracted
   b. Loss of DIP joint flexion may not be noted initially because of partial compensation from intact flexor digitorum superficialis tendon; thus, avulsed tendon must be isolated when testing flexor strength
   c. Pain and swelling
3. Treatment
   a. With early diagnosis (< 3 wks), tendon can usually be repaired surgically
   b. After 6 wks, primary surgical repair not possible, and DIP fusion or reconstruction attempted

DIP Joint Dislocation

1. Mechanism of Injury: dorsal and often open
2. Treatment
   a. Stable reduction easily accomplished on field by applying adequate traction and bringing bones out to length
   b. Immobilize joint for 3 wks and then protect during competition for 2–3 wks

INJURIES TO THE PROXIMAL INTERPHALANGEAL (PIP) JOINT

The "Jammed" Finger

1. Mechanism of Injury: longitudinally directed force applied to extended PIP joint
2. Clinical Presentation: localized tenderness
3. Physical Examination
   a. Assess central extensor tendon insertion rupture by extending finger against resistance
   b. Test volar plate integrity by hyperextending PIP joint and comparing extension to adjacent normal PIP joint
   c. Assess collateral ligament integrity by stressing extended joint in medial-lateral direction
   d. Pain and swelling may persist for 3–6 mos
3. Radiographic Evaluation: obtain AP and lateral views to rule out bone injury
4. Treatment
   a. After inflammation subsides, warm soaks and buddy tape to adjacent normal finger
   b. Buddy tape for competition as long as joint sore

Articular Fractures

1. Mechanism of Injury
   a. Can involve either proximal phalanx condyles (Fig. 15–7) or middle phalanx articular base
   b. Forcible hyperextension or acute flexion against resistance causes avulsion fractures of base of middle phalanx
2. Treatment
   a. Treat nondisplaced or minimally displaced fractures (ie, < 2 mm displacement) conservatively
      (1) Splint PIP joint in no more than 30° flexion
      (2) Immobilize MCP joint of injured finger and adjacent finger, especially if rotational and angular instability possible
      (3) 3–4 wks of splinting usually necessary to minimize risk of displacement

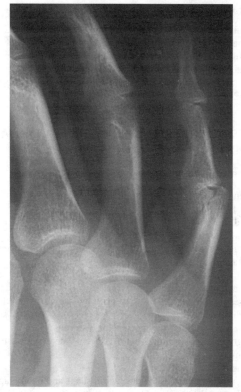

Fig. 15–7. Condylar fracture of the PIP joint.

b. Comminuted fractures or very small fracture fragments best treated by closed reduction and splinting; initiate joint exercises within 2–3 wks
c. Surgery indicated for large, displaced fractures
d. Splint dorsal fractures with PIP joint in full extension; splint volar fractures with PIP joint in 25° flexion
   (1) Surgery indicated when fracture involves more than ⅓ of articular surface, displacement > 3 mm, or PIP joint subluxation
   (2) Remove splint 2–3 wks after injury or surgery and protectively exercise finger; at 4 wks, start passive mobilization
   (3) Use protective splints and buddy tape for early return to competition

Fracture-Dislocations

1. Mechanism of Injury
   a. Dorsal dislocation with small volar plate avulsion fracture (Fig. 15–8)
   b. Longitudinally directed force applied to extended PIP joint (same mechanism as jammed finger)
2. Clinical Presentation: same as for jammed finger
3. Radiographic Evaluation
   a. Lateral view shows volar lip fracture of middle phalanx with dorsal dislocation of middle phalanx
   b. Collateral ligament avulsion fractures also possible
4. Treatment
   a. Reduce dislocation by applying longitudinal traction to finger (ideally, perform under local or regional anesthesia to assess joint stability and ligament integrity)
   b. Splint PIP joint initially in approximately 60° flexion

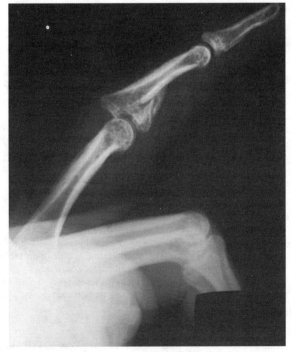

Fig. 15–8. Dorsal fracture-dislocation of the PIP joint.

    c. Follow with extension block splinting, extending joint about 15°
   each wk until full extension possible (usually within 4–6 wks)

    d. During athletic activity, buddy tape affected finger for 2–3 wks

    e. If joint stable, further treatment depends on fracture pattern

    f. Surgery indicated if fracture comminuted or if injury involves
   more than 35–40% of articular surface

    g. If collateral ligament lax, immediate surgical repair indicated

    h. After surgery, splint finger at 25° flexion for 2–3 wks, then start
   gentle active exercises

    i. No full extension until 4 wks after surgery; during interim, exten-
   sion block splinting may be used

PIP Joint Dislocations

1. Mechanism of Injury

    a. May be dorsal, lateral, or volar

    b. Dorsal dislocation (most common) caused by hyperextension (Fig.
   15–9)

    c. Volar plate disrupted and accessory collateral ligaments tear, but
   collateral ligaments often not affected

2. Radiographic Evaluation: rule out associated fractures

3. Treatment

    a. If no coexisting fractures, reduce dislocated PIP joint by accen-
   tuating deformity and then applying traction to finger while flexing it

    b. For uncomplicated dorsal dislocation without collateral ligament
   damage, splint finger with PIP joint at 25–30° flexion for 2–3
   wks, then start gentle ROM exercises; buddy tape until full painless motion possible

    c. Treat dorsal dislocation with collateral ligament injury, lateral
   dislocation of PIP joint (where single collateral ligament ruptures),
   and volar disruption of PIP joint surgically

Injuries to the Collateral Ligaments

1. Mechanism of Injury: isolated collateral ligament injury (eg,
   ''sprained'' finger)

2. Clinical Presentation: joint tenderness and swelling

3. Treatment

    a. Splint partial tears, or those with only mild laxity and good end
   point in slight flexion until pain abates; buddy tape or protectively
   splint during activity until full painless motion returns

    b. Repair all complete tears surgically; after surgery, splint finger
   in slight flexion for 3 wks, then start motion exercises

Boutonnière Deformity

1. Mechanism of Injury

    a. Either severe flexion force or direct blow to dorsal PIP joint

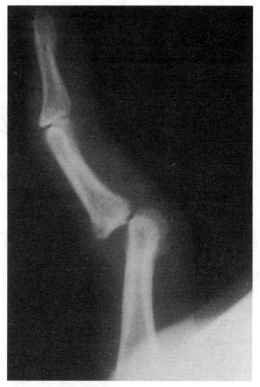

Fig. 15–9. Dorsal dislocation of the PIP joint.

    b. Develops after failure to diagnose and treat avulsion or fracture
       of central slip on middle phalanx
2. Clinical Presentation
    a. Fixed PIP joint flexion with fixed DIP joint hyperextension (Fig.
       15-10)
    b. Inability to extend PIP joint
3. Treatment
    a. Splint finger with PIP joint in full extension
       (1) May need 3 mos or more of splinting
       (2) Continue night splinting and splinting during activities for 2
           more months
    b. Surgery indicated for chronic deformity

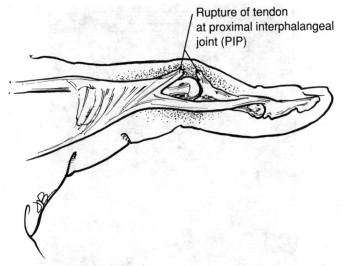

Fig. 15–10. Classic boutonnière deformity: fixed flexion of the PIP joint with fixed hyperextension of the DIP joint.

Pseudoboutonnière Deformity

1. Mechanism of Injury
   a. Follows hyperextension injury to PIP joint in response to volar plate rupture
   b. Central slip not injured
2. Clinical Presentation: PIP joint flexion contracture with slight DIP joint hyperextension that is not fixed, permitting active flexion
3. Radiographic Evaluation: calcification at proximal attachment of PIP volar plate
4. Treatment
   a. Treat mild deformities (ie, PIP joint flexion contracture < 40°) nonsurgically with dynamic extension or "safety pin" splint to passively improve PIP joint extension
   b. Reserve surgery for flexion contracture > 40°; maintain finger in extension for 3 wks after surgery

Injuries to the Volar Plate

1. Mechanism of Injury: PIP joint hyperextension may disrupt volar plate without frank joint dislocation
2. Clinical Presentation
   a. Swollen PIP joint and tenderness over palmar joint; finger slightly flexed

b. Pain, swelling, and guarding may limit demonstrating acute hyperextension
3. Treatment
   a. Immobilize joint in slight flexion for 2–3 wks; then start active exercises with interim protective splinting
   b. If full extension slow to return, initiate passive stretching at 4 wks

INJURIES TO THE METACARPOPHALANGEAL (MCP) JOINT

General Treatment Protocol

1. Splint in at least 45° flexion, and preferably in 70°
2. As flexion increases, collateral ligaments tighten, bony contact of joint surfaces increases, and joint becomes more stable
3. If joint immobilized in extension, healing supporting structures contract and seriously limit flexion when movement initiated

Dislocations

1. Mechanism of Injury
   a. Forced finger hyperextension can cause dorsal dislocation (Fig. 15–11)

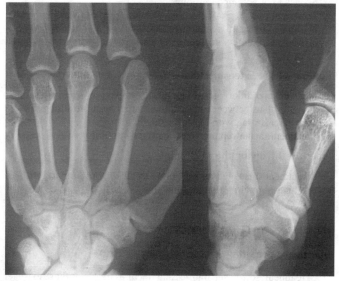

Fig. 15–11. Dislocation of the MCP joint.

   b. Normally, volar plate ruptures proximally and remains attached to proximal plate
2. Incomplete or ''Simple'' Dislocation
   a. Clinical Presentation: volar plate not interposed in joint and MCP joint usually fixed in hyperextension
   b. Treatment
      (1) Do not apply longitudinal traction, which may result in complex, irreducible dislocation with volar plate interposed in joint
      (2) Reduce dislocation by holding joint surfaces in contact while accentuating deformity, flexing wrist to reduce tension on flexor tendons, and gently manipulating joint into place
3. Complex Dislocation
   a. Clinical Presentation
      (1) Characteristic dimple in palm
      (2) Joint not fixed in grossly hyperextended position
      (3) Ulnar deviation of injured finger
   b. Treatment: open reduction usually necessary

Injuries to the Collateral Ligaments

1. Mechanism of Injury: lateral deviation of flexed MCP joint with collateral ligaments under tension
2. Radiographic Evaluation: make sure avulsion fracture from metacarpal head not entrapped in joint
3. Treatment
   a. Buddy tape until symptoms resolve
   b. May need surgery in chronic cases where ligament ends interposed in joint

Rupture of the Extensor Hood

1. Mechanism of Injury: hood rupture allows extensor tendon to subluxate into sulcus between adjacent metacarpal heads, resulting in MCP joint extensor lag with loss of strength
2. Treatment: acute ruptures best managed surgically

Fractures Involving the MCP Joint

   Treatment: managed as PIP joint fractures, with primary goals of maintaining normal motion and function

INJURIES TO THE THUMB

Interphalangeal Joint

   Treatment: soft-tissue injuries and fractures treated as those to finger PIP joints

Dislocation of the MCP Joint

1. Mechanism of Injury
   a. Dorsal dislocation similar to that of MCP joints of fingers
   b. Volar plate may tear proximally or distally
2. Treatment: Closed reduction by gentle manipulation possible, but open reduction often necessary to ensure stability

Injuries to the Ulnar Collateral Ligament of the MCP Joint

1. Mechanism of Injury
   a. Abduction stress applied to thumb while MCP joint near full extension (Fig. 15–12)
   b. Skeletally mature athletes disrupt ligament, whereas skeletally immature athletes fracture proximal phalanx
2. Radiographic Evaluation: ligament avulsion off ulnar proximal phalanx
3. Physical Examination

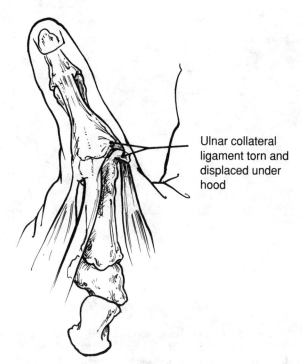

Ulnar collateral ligament torn and displaced under hood

Fig. 15–12. Avulsion of the ulnar collateral ligament.

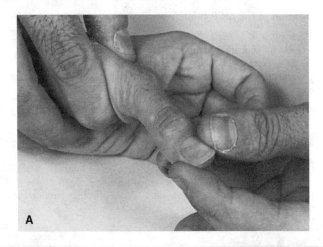

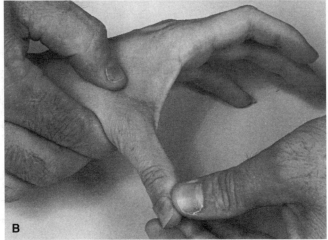

Fig. 15–13. Stress testing of the ulnar collateral ligament with the thumb in slight flexion (A) and in full extension (B).

a. If radiographs negative, assess ligament integrity by comparing with uninjured thumb
b. Stress MCP joint in full extension and in 30° flexion (Fig. 15–13)
c. Radial deviation > 25–30° indicates at least partial tear
d. Lack of firm end point, particularly in full extension, indicates complete tear

e. Thumb displays hyperextension laxity if volar plate and accessory collateral ligaments also injured
4. Treatment
    a. Immobilize partial tears in thumb spica cast
    b. Complete tears require surgical repair
    c. In both cases, immobilize thumb in 20° flexion for 3 wks; leave IP joint free to permit active motion and prevent scarring of extensor mechanism
    d. At 3–4 wks, use removable splint and start active exercises; remove splint after 5–6 wks and return to activity
    e. During activity, protect thumb for 3 mos by buddy taping or silicone cast

Injuries to the Radial Collateral Ligament of the MCP Joint

1. Mechanism of Injury: volar subluxation of proximal phalanx
2. Treatment: similar to ulnar collateral ligament injury, with intent of preventing further volar subluxation or laxity of radial side of joint

Injuries to the Carpometacarpal (CMC) Joint of the Thumb

1. Bennett's fracture
    a. Mechanism of Injury: forcible thumb abduction results in oblique intra-articular fracture at CMC joint base that transects proximal articular surface
    b. Treatment
        (1) Closed reduction may work for nondisplaced or minimally displaced fractures
        (2) If displacement persists, closed reduction and external fixation may be needed; or ORIF
2. Fracture-Dislocation
    a. Mechanism of Injury: rare, but may occur with severe force exerted against hyperextended hand
    b. Treatment: closed reduction; however, with associated interposition of soft tissue and tendons, ORIF required
3. Complete Dislocation
    a. Mechanism of Injury
        (1) Rare without concomitant fracture
        (2) Fall on outstretched hand with hyperabduction or hyperextension forces directed across volar metacarpal bone
    b. Treatment
        (1) In most cases, acute dislocations easily reduced
        (2) Immobilize joint in either long- or short-arm thumb spica cast for 3 wks, followed by 3 more wks in short-arm thumb spica cast; then start active exercise
        (3) For chronic instability or subluxation, open reduction and repair of volar ligament

FRACTURES TO THE SHAFT OF THE FINGERS

Phalangeal Fractures

1. Treatment
   a. Splint undisplaced fractures with MCP joint in 70° flexion and IP joints in slight flexion
   b. Manipulate displaced fractures into position and then immobilize as above

Metacarpal Fractures

1. Mechanism of Injury: direct trauma or crushing injury
2. Evaluation
   a. Degree of angulation determined only by radiographs
   b. Assess rotational deformity clinically by individually flexing each finger into palm; any deviation from point to scaphoid indicates rotational deformity
3. Treatment
   a. Treat acute metacarpal neck fractures by closed reduction, correcting any rotational deformity
   b. Splint finger with MCP and IP joints in 45° flexion with finger tip pointed toward scaphoid
   c. Splint oblique or spiral fractures anteriorly for 2–3 wks
   d. Multiple fractures may require ORIF

NEUROCOMPRESSIVE INJURIES TO THE HAND

1. Mechanism of Injury: persistent, repetitive, controlled stress
2. Acute Injuries
   a. Mechanical or 2° to ischemic insult
   b. Powerful force compresses nerve against unyielding structure
   c. Injury normally isolated and transitory
3. Chronic Injuries
   a. Predictable sites
   b. May affect either median nerve in carpal tunnel or ulnar nerve in Guyon's canal
4. Clinical Presentation
   a. Compression of Median Nerve
      (1) Paresthesia in thumb, index, or long fingers, and subsequent thenar muscle atrophy
      (2) Elicit symptoms by tapping over nerve (Tinel's sign) at wrist or by prolonged flexion of wrist (Phalen's sign)
   b. Compression of Ulnar Nerve
      (1) Ulnar neuropathy with possible distal sensory changes
      (2) Painful mass at thumb base

5. Treatment
- a. Median Nerve
  - (1) Conservative treatment: rest and NSAIDs
  - (2) Reserve surgery for unresponsive cases
- b. Ulnar Nerve: correct underlying cause

Hip Injuries

FRACTURES OF THE PELVIS

Fractures of the Ilium

1. Mechanism of Injury
   a. Backward fall
   b. May be pelvic viscera damage and retroperitoneal hemorrhage with preservation of ring's integrity
2. Clinical Presentation
   a. Immediate pain prevents ambulation
   b. Pelvic tenderness, swelling posteriorly, and ecchymosis
3. Radiographic Evaluation: To evaluate bone injury
4. Treatment
   a. Conservative treatment: bed rest until acute pain ↓
   b. Restrict activity until pain ↓; use support or taping as activities resumed
   c. Protected weight bearing with crutches for 2–3 wks
   d. Return to competition restricted for 3–4 mos

Fractures of the Sacrum

1. Mechanism of Injury
   a. Fall in sitting position or direct blow
   b. Distal fragment angulates forward and becomes impacted
2. Clinical Presentation
   a. Severe pain
   b. Sacral tenderness (rectal examination pinpoints tenderness anteriorly)
3. Radiographic Evaluation: radiographs and MRI identify lesion
4. Treatment
   a. Bed rest followed by protected weight bearing
   b. Surgery necessary only if fracture fragments significantly displaced, which could injure sacral nerve roots and cause bladder paralysis

Fractures of the Coccyx

1. Mechanism of Injury
   a. Fall in sitting position

    b. Fracture may occur at sacrococcygeal junction or in coccygeal body
2. Clinical Presentation
    a. Severe pain at time of injury, during sudden movements, and while sitting
    b. Coccygeal tenderness (rectal examination pinpoints tenderness and painful motion of coccyx)
3. Radiographic Evaluation: lateral view reveals lesion
4. Treatment
    a. Directed at relieving pain
        (1) Sitting forward with weight distributed on ischial tuberosities frees coccyx of posterior pressure
        (2) Avoid tight undergarments or pants
        (3) Lying supine relieves pressure on bone
    b. Coccyx may remain chronically painful and tender, but excision not recommended
    c. Return to athletic activity as soon as comfort allows

Fractures of the Acetabulum

1. Mechanism of Injury: direct violent force through femoral neck into acetabulum
2. Clinical Presentation
    a. Immediate pain and inability to walk on leg
    b. Pain with passive or active hip ROM
    c. Extremity shortening due to central acetabular displacement
3. Radiographic Evaluation: to determine extent of fracture
4. Treatment
    a. Bed rest, followed by ROM for both displaced and nondisplaced fractures until pain subsides and healing occurs
    b. Protected weight bearing with crutches
    c. Skeletal traction or ORIF may be needed to reduce some displaced fractures

TRAUMATIC DISLOCATION OF THE HIP

General Principles

1. True medical emergency in which early reduction important to prevent avascular necrosis
2. Do not attempt to reduce on the field

Posterior Dislocation

1. Mechanism of Injury
    a. Impact forces femoral head posteriorly, tearing ligamentum teres and posterior capsule (Fig. 16–1)
    b. Posterior acetabulum may be fractured, vascular supply to femoral head disrupted, and sciatic nerve injured

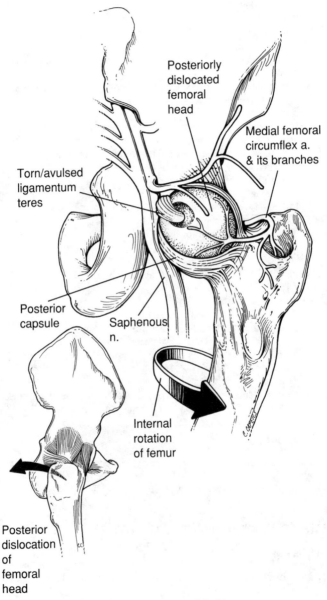

Fig. 16–1. Diagram of a posterior dislocation of the hip.

2. Clinical Presentation
   a. Pain
   b. Limb held in internal rotation as hip flexed and adducted
3. Physical Examination
   a. Have patient dorsiflex foot to evaluate peroneal division of sciatic nerve
   b. Have patient plantar flex and invert foot to evaluate tibial portion of sciatic nerve
4. Treatment
   a. Closed reduction usually requires adequate analgesia or general anesthesia
   b. If dislocation recurs, open reduction may be needed
   c. After reduction, place limb in traction suspension
   d. Start ROM early and ambulate with crutches approximately 2 wks after injury
   e. Protected weight bearing for 2–6 mos
   f. If surgery necessary, protect for 6 wks
   g. No return to athletics for at least 3 mos

Anterior Dislocation

1. Mechanism of Injury: forceful abduction and external rotation (Fig.16-2)
2. Clinical Presentation
   a. Pain
   b. Abducted and externally rotated limb
   c. Palpable groin mass
   d. Displaced femoral head can compress femoral vein and produce thrombus
3. Treatment
   a. Closed reduction usually accomplished under general anesthesia with longitudinal traction and internal rotation of extremity
   b. Open reduction rarely required

Central Dislocation

1. Mechanism of Injury: femoral head protrusion into fractured acetabulum
2. Treatment: as for fractured acetabulum

SLIPPED CAPITAL FEMORAL EPIPHYSIS

Mechanism of Injury

1. Not always identifiable because weakened growth plate subject to fracture from normal stresses

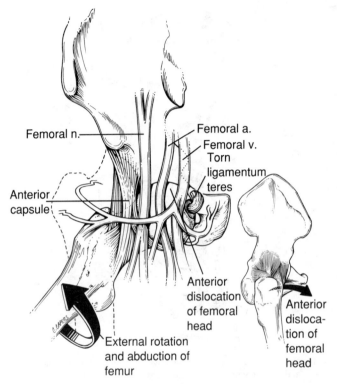

Fig. 16–2. Diagram of an anterior dislocation of the hip.

2. Femoral neck rotates anteriorly and laterally, while head slips posteriorly and medially (Fig. 16–3)
3. Rate of slippage can be fast (acute) or slow (chronic)

Clinical Presentation

Pain may be referred to knee
Gluteus medius limp

Radiographic Evaluation: diagnose by femoral neck radiographic appearance

Treatment

1. Depends on type and degree of slip
2. Perform ORIF as soon as possible to prevent further displacement and avascular necrosis

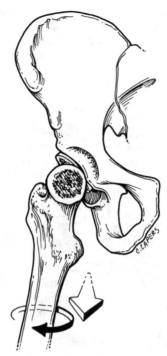

Fig. 16–3. In slipped capital femoral epiphysis, the femoral neck rotates anterior and laterad, while the head goes posterior and mediad.

FRACTURES OF THE PROXIMAL FEMUR

Mechanism of Injury

1. Intracapsular fractures: indirect forces, such as shear force on angulated femoral neck
2. Extracapsular fractures: direct trauma to hip

Clinical Presentation

1. Intracapsular Fractures
   a. Immediate pain
   b. If fracture displaced, leg may be shortened and externally rotated
   c. If impacted or nondisplaced, deformity minimal
   d. Pain with ROM most consistent sign
2. Extracapsular Fractures
   a. May be comminuted with significant blood loss

b. Immediate pain and inability to walk

c. More pronounced external rotation and shortening of leg

Treatment

1. ORIF for both types of fractures
2. Applying traction to extremity relieves pain during transfer

OVERUSE INJURIES OF THE HIP

Stress Fractures of the Femoral Neck

1. Mechanism of Injury
   a. If no underlying bone disease, then history of increase or change in training
   b. Untreated simple stress fracture may progress to displaced femoral neck fracture
2. Clinical Presentation
   a. "Achy" pain localized to anterior groin or thigh
   b. Prominent morning symptoms often relieved by moderate activity
   c. Athlete may not notice significant hip pain until middle of training run
   d. ↓ motion and pain at extremes of flexion and internal rotation may be subtle
   e. Tenderness to palpation not prominent
3. Radiographic Evaluation
   a. Normal radiographs do not show characteristic sclerosis and subtle fracture line until several wks after onset of symptoms (Fig. 16–4)
   b. Standard diagnostic test: radioisotope bone scan
   c. If radiographs and bone scan negative, use MRI to confirm diagnosis
4. Treatment
   a. Stress Reactions and Compression Side Stress Fractures
      (1) Treat with protected weight bearing until morning pain eliminated and painless ambulation possible
      (2) Water exercises and stationary cycling maintain aerobic capacity during healing
      (3) Gradually ↑ pain-free activity until repetitive loading painless
      (4) Restrict activity for 6–8 wks and curtail if pain recurs
      (5) Full recovery may take 2 yrs or longer
   b. Tension Side Stress Fractures
      (1) Treat surgically to prevent complications of fracture displacement
      (2) Restrict athletic activity until radiographic evidence of healing
   c. Displaced Stress Fractures of the Femoral Neck: closed reduction or ORIF

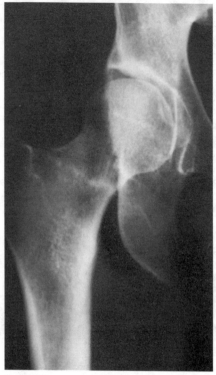

Fig. 16–4. This medial compression type stress fracture of the femoral neck demonstrates the typical sclerosis and endosteal callus seen 2 to 4 weeks after onset of symptoms.

Other Stress Fractures

1. Pubic Ramus Stress Fractures
   a. Mechanism of Injury
      (1) Tensile stresses generated in hamstring muscle origins
      (2) Bilateral lesions or development of contralateral fracture common
   b. Treatment: restrict painful activities
2. Stress Fractures of the Femoral Shaft
   a. Mechanism of Injury: significant compressive stresses generated in medial subtrochanteric region
   b. Radiographic Evaluation: medial cortex thickening of femur and occasionally fracture line
   c. Treatment: restrict painful activities

Pain at Muscle Origins

1. Adult Athletes
   a. Proximal adductor musculature strain: most common painful overuse injury about hip
   b. Abductor musculature may also be strained
   c. Tendinitis of gluteus medius origin near iliac crest can cause painful disability
   d. Treatment: after initial pain subsides, heat or ultrasound, gentle stretching, NSAIDs, and progressive resistance exercises
2. "Growing" Adolescent Athletes

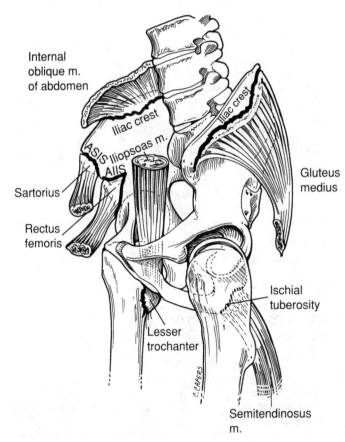

Fig. 16–5. Common sites of avulsion injuries of the hip in adolescents.

a. Tend to injure apophyses, where pelvic girdle musculature originates, rather than muscles or tendons themselves (Fig. 16–5)
b. Mechanism of Injury
  (1) Muscle attachments fail due to sudden muscle loading, or more gradually, with repetitive stress (apophysitis)
  (2) "Hip pointer": avulsion of iliac apophysis from pelvis by strong contraction of abdominal musculature or direct blow
c. Diagnosis based on history, physical examination, and characteristic radiographic changes
d. Treatment of Apophysitis
  (1) Protect from loading during healing, usually by protected weight bearing with crutches
  (2) Surgery not necessary
  (3) Stretching involved muscle groups prevents excessive tension on apophysis
  (4) Gradual return to activity as dictated by pain
  (5) In rare cases, may need to remove displaced apophysis or mass of ectopic bone that forms during healing
  (6) Padding apophysis during contact sports may prevent reinjury
  (7) Restrict full return to activity until flexibility and strength regained

BURSITIS AND THE SNAPPING HIP

Trochanteric Bursitis

1. Chronic inflammation of bursa between gluteus maximus-tensor fascia lata muscles and greater trochanter of femur
2. Diagnosed by direct palpation and sometimes by injection of local anesthetic
3. Treatment
  a. Eliminate activity that causes pain
  b. Stretch iliotibial band in flexion and extension
  c. NSAIDs or local corticosteroid injections

BURSITIS OF THE ILIOPSOAS BURSA
Can Cause Groin Pain in Athletes

External Snapping Hip

1. Caused by chronic bursitis or fibrosis of gluteus maximus
2. Clinical Presentation
  a. Sensation of clunking or subluxation in hip while walking, running, or pivoting
  b. Elicit symptomatic snap by extending knee and hip in adduction and then flexing hip

    c. Patient can demonstrate snapping while standing with hip extended and forcibly internally rotating it
3. Treatment
    a. Treat underlying bursitis
    b. Treat surgically resistant cases with fibrosis of underlying structures

Internal Snapping Hip

1. Caused by secondary tendinitis and chronic bursitis of iliopsoas bursa
2. Iliopsoas tendon snaps over iliopectineal eminence where it crosses pelvic brim, usually when hip extends from flexed, abducted, externally rotated position
3. Snapping sensation associated with pain in deep anterior groin
4. Treatment
    a. Stretch hip flexor musculature
    b. Resistant cases may be treated surgically

INGUINAL HERNIA

Mechanism of Injury

Extrusion of portion of abdominal contents through abdominal wall defect

Clinical Presentation

Anterior groin pain

Treatment

Surgical correction, with return to activity by 3 mos after surgery

Musculotendinous Injuries About the Knee

MUSCLE STRAINS

Mechanism of Injury

1. Forcefully contracting muscle subjected to strong passive force in opposite direction
2. Rapid stretching of active muscle beyond optimal length disrupts or permanently weakens parts of myotendinous junction

Classification

1. Grade I: Low-grade inflammatory response with minimal structural damage
2. Grade II: Actual tissue damage
3. Grade III: Complete disruption of some portion of musculotendinous unit, but not complete rupture

Clinical Presentation

1. Grade I
   a. Soreness or tightness in injured area
   b. With hamstrings strains, tightness during extreme hip flexion, but resisted knee flexion generally pain free
   c. No pain to palpation and no swelling or change in thigh girth
   d. Unchanged gait cycle and normal hip ROM
   e. Diagnose quadriceps strain with < 90° ROM in prone position with hip fully extended and minimal loss of strength
2. Grade II
   a. Athlete may report feeling or hearing "pop" in posterior thigh (hamstring) region during activity
   b. Swelling and ↑ thigh girth with both quadriceps and hamstrings strains
   c. Painful palpation of muscle defect
   d. Pain resulting in abnormal gait
      (1) Quadriceps Strains
         (a) Reluctance to flex knee when walking

(b) Using hip adductors to pull leg through swing phase of gait, causing external rotation at hip

(2) Hamstrings Strains

(a) Knee flexed while walking to minimize pain of full extension

(b) Limited hip flexion, even with knee flexed, causes hamstring shortening

e. Quadriceps strains compromise strength

3. Grade III

a. Severe pain at time of injury

b. Sound or feel of ''pop'' in hamstring region

c. Swelling and significant ↑ in thigh girth

d. Palpable muscle defects or masses

e. ↓ strength

f. With hamstrings strains, passive hip flexion or knee extension causes pain

Treatment

1. Starts with RICE: rest, ice, compression, and elevation

a. Rest ranges from temporary cessation of sports to avoidance of weight bearing using crutches

b. Crushed ice in bag conforms to injured area; hold in place with compression dressing and ice 2–3 times daily for 15–20 min per session

2. NSAIDs to reduce swelling and pain in acute injuries

3. Progression of treatment depends on injury severity, pain, and ability to perform functional activities

4. Grade I strains usually evident within 48 hrs, but may take up to 1 wk to identify Grade II or III strains

5. Evaluate pain, thigh girth, injury site, pain-free arc of knee motion, and muscle testing daily

6. Progress rehab from isometric to isotonic to isokinetic exercises, with pain as guide

Return to Activity

1. Grade I: No lost competition or practice time

2. Grade II: 1–3 wks of lost competition or practice time

3. Grade III: 3 wks to 3 mos of lost competition or practice time

QUADRICEPS CONTUSION/HEMATOMA

Mechanism of Injury

1. Blunt trauma to anterior thigh causes bleeding deep within muscle and between muscle planes

2. Compression wave generated within quadriceps travels through su-

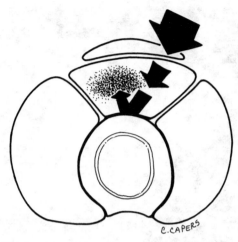

Fig. 17-1. Drawing shows motion of compression wave, causing quadriceps contusion.

perficial musculature, but cannot be transmitted through incompressible bone, causing crushing of vastus intermedius against femur (Fig. 17-1)

Classification

1. Mild: > 90° active knee motion 12-24 hrs after injury
2. Moderate: 45-90°
3. Severe: < 45°

Clinical Presentation

1. Swelling and pain
2. ↓ knee ROM
3. Knee stiffness

Treatment

1. Ice bags and compression wraps with knee immobilized in maximum flexion
2. Serial distal vascular and neurologic examinations for 48 hrs
3. Measure thigh girth at intervals to monitor any progression of bleeding
4. If within 8 hrs of injury, aspirate hematoma and inject with 1% Xylocaine, corticosteroid, and hyaluronidase
5. Once thigh girth stabilizes, start rehab
6. ROM exercises, weight bearing as tolerated, and ice massage with gravity-assisted motion in flexion and extension

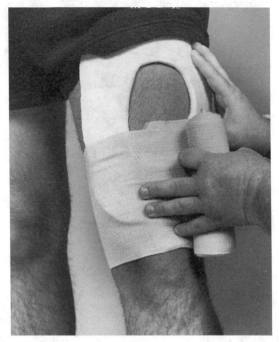

Fig. 17–2. Thigh pads or doughnut pads are used to protect a quadriceps contusion.

7. Never use heat during treatment, as it ↑ risk of rebleeding
8. When pain-free active knee flexion exceeds 120°, start functional rehab, with return to activity when ROM is full
9. Extra-large thigh pads or doughnut pads held in place with neoprene sleeves or elastic wraps provide added protection of contused area (Fig. 17–2)

ACUTE COMPARTMENT SYNDROME

Mechanism of Injury

Quadriceps contusion causes such severe swelling that pressure in unyielding fascial sheath results in reduced capillary blood flow and neuromuscular compromise

Clinical Presentation

1. Can develop as early as few hrs or as late as 64 hrs after injury
2. Primary sign: pain out of proportion to injury

3. If seen late, weak knee extension, pain on passive knee flexion, and altered sensation over knee and medial leg and foot (these findings may be absent, however, even with high intracompartmental pressures)

Diagnostic Modalities

1. Measure intracompartmental pressure by Whitesides' technique, wick catheter, slit catheter, or infusion method
2. Pressure ≥ 30mm Hg indicates need for prompt surgical intervention
3. Laboratory studies: hemoglobin, hematocrit, electrolytes, PT, PTT, and platelet counts

Treatment

1. Surgical emergency (irreversible injury can occur within 5–6 hrs of onset of ischemia): perform fasciotomy
2. Postoperative rehab depends on size of fasciotomy wound and amount of necrosis
3. Return to activity depends on initial contusion and severity of compartment damage

MYOSITIS OSSIFICANS TRAUMATICA

Mechanism of Injury

1. Benign, localized formation of heterotopic non-neoplastic bone results from physical trauma to muscles near bone
2. Severe compression of muscles and other soft tissues against bone causes disruption of muscle fibers, connective tissue, blood vessels, and periosteum

Clinical Presentation

1. Suspect if local pain, swelling, and tenderness of quadriceps contusion do not respond to conservative treatment within 4–5 days of injury
2. Very probable if local symptoms have not improved significantly within 2 wks, if symptoms ↑ during this time, or if induration becomes more pronounced

Radiographic Evaluation

1. Initially, no radiographic evidence
2. By 3–4 wks, flocculent densities arise within muscle and periosteal reaction may be present in underlying bone
3. By 6–8 wks, sharply circumscribed lacy pattern of new bone visible about mass edges (ossification not seen in central core of mass)(Fig. 17–3)
4. Maturing lesion becomes more dense and occasionally attaches directly to bone

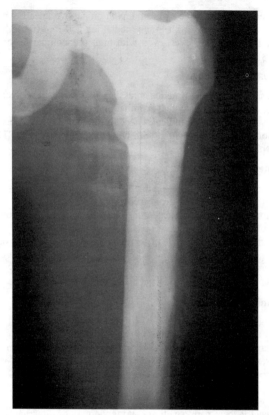

Fig. 17–3. Radiograph of early-stage myositis ossificans.

5. Lesion reaches maximum size at 6 mos (Fig. 17–4) and then shrinks over several mos
6. Three-phase bone scan, arteriography, ultrasonography, CT, and MRI can be used to evaluate lesion

Treatment

1. Acute management similar to that for moderate to severe quadriceps contusion
   a. RICE, immobilization, and limited weight bearing
   b. Aspirate hematoma and inject with 1% Xylocaine, steroid, and hyaluronidase if seen within 8 hrs of injury
2. Oral indomethacin, 50 mg t.i.d.

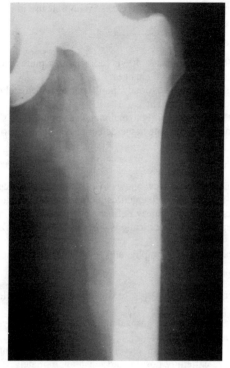

Fig. 17–4. Radiograph of late-stage myositis ossificans.

3. Rehab protocol as for quadriceps contusion, using pain and ROM to guide progression and return to activity
4. Pad to protect injured area from repeated trauma
5. Surgical removal of lesion
   a. May be indicated for persistent local pain or muscle dysfunction or if limited adjacent joint ROM results in functional disability
   b. Do not consider until at least 6 mos after injury to ensure lesion maturity

QUADRICEPS TENDON RUPTURE

Mechanism of Injury

1. Complete rupture due to sudden, violent quadriceps contraction, usually from fall

2. Microscopic partial tears 2° to excessive muscle use in weight room, as with squats

Clinical Presentation

1. Almost 90% of patients > 40 yrs old: tendon ruptures thought 2° to age-related degenerative changes
2. Frequently, athlete hears loud "pop" and is immediately unable to extend leg or bear weight
3. Complete rupture: inability to maintain knee in full extension against gravity and palpable soft tissue defect proximal to superior patellar pole

Radiographic Evaluation

1. Lateral radiographic view shows loss of normal quadriceps outline and soft-tissue mass with calcification representing retracted tendon
2. Other abnormalities: poorly defined suprapatellar mass, obliterated quadriceps tendon, calcifications, patella baja, joint effusion, and patellar spurring
3. CT, ultrasound, arthrography, and MRI may help

Treatment

1. Microscopic partial tears resolve rapidly if causative factors discontinued
2. Tendon ruptures require surgical intervention (conservative treatment results in poor outcomes)
3. For best results, perform surgery as soon as possible after injury, immobilize extremity postop, and rehab appropriately
4. Residual problems: patellar pain, loss of quadriceps strength, residual extension lag, and myositis ossificans of quadriceps tendon

RUPTURE OF THE PATELLAR TENDON

Mechanism of Injury

1. "Noncontact" injury (from pivoting, twisting, or deceleration) rather than direct trauma
2. Associated vulnerable structures: extracapsular structures, ACL, and medial or lateral stabilizing structures (eg, MCL)

Clinical Presentation

1. Palpable defect in patellar tendon and patella alta (knee must be flexed 90° during examination)
2. Gap of > 1 fingerbreadth between inferior patellar pole and joint line (patella alta) suggests rupture of infrapatellar tendon

Radiographic Evaluation

1. Plain radiography may outline patella alta
2. If not detected within 2 wks, significant proximal patellar retraction may develop, with quadriceps contracture and adhesions

Treatment: Surgical Repair

JUMPER'S KNEE

Mechanism of Injury

1. Overuse insertional tendinitis of quadriceps (at upper patellar pole) and patellar tendon (at lower pole)
2. Affects athletes who expose knees to continuous stresses and eccentric efforts that exceed intrinsic tensile resistance of extensor mechanism
3. Sudden and repeated overload of knee extensor mechanism, sometimes aggravated by imbalance within mechanism, weakens tendon structures
4. Overload occurs when athlete lands on leg with knee semiflexed; when foot leaves ground after eccentric contraction phase of quadriceps; or in acceleration, deceleration, stopping, or cutting movements

Classification

1. Level 1: No pain
2. Level 2: Pain with extreme exertion only
3. Level 3: Pain with exertion and 1–2 hrs after
4. Level 4: Pain during any athletic activity and 4–6 hrs after, plus ↓ performance
5. Level 5: Pain immediately after beginning sports activity and withdrawal from activity
6. Level 6: Pain during daily activities and inability to participate in any sports

Clinical Presentation

1. Pain anteriorly, most often at tendinous insertion on lower patellar pole
2. Pain exacerbated by physical activity or prolonged sitting with knee flexed
3. Quadriceps atrophy, vastus medialis obliquus (VMO) dysplasia, and functional insufficiency of flexor dorsalis of ankle
4. No joint swelling

Physical Examination

1. Elicit pain by palpating tendinous insertion on lower or upper patellar pole or (less often) over tendon belly or tibial tuberosity
2. Pain exacerbated by sudden quadriceps contraction, passive knee flexion > 120°, squatting, and resisted leg extension

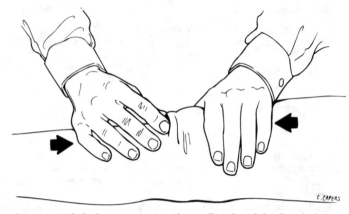

C.CAPERS

Fig. 17–5. With the knee in extension, the patella is forced distally, which slightly elevates the distal pole. The distal pole is then palpated for tenderness.

3. With knee extended, distal pole elevates slightly when patella forced distally (Fig. 17–5).
4. Meniscal tests negative

Radiographic Evaluation

1. Lateral radiograph using soft-tissue technique shows
   a. Thick tendon belly
   b. Degeneration
   c. Occasionally, elongations or irregularities of distal patellar pole
   d. Ossicles in tendon
2. Ultrasonography, CT, and MRI can help

Treatment

1. Levels 1–5 Injuries
   a. Conservative treatment: rest, continue activities within limits of symptoms, NSAIDs, cryotherapy, and other physical therapy modalities
   b. Avoid intratendinous corticosteroid injection because of risk of rupture
   c. Progress rehab from isometric to isotonic to isokinetic exercises, with pain as guide
   d. Wear infrapatellar band to reduce stress on tendon insertion (Fig. 17-6)
2. Level 6 Injury
   a. Conservative treatment, but with longer period of rest from any activity that causes pain

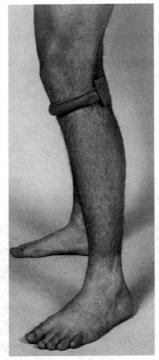

Fig. 17–6. The infrapatellar band can be worn to reduce stress on the tendon insertion.

    b. If no improvement after 4–6 mos, surgery indicated
3. Complete Rupture or Avulsion of the Tendon: Requires surgical intervention

OSGOOD-SCHLATTER DISEASE

Mechanism of Injury

1. Apophysitis of tibial tubercle at patellar tendon insertion
2. Functional overload from repetitive stresses on patellar tendon or direct trauma to tibial tuberosity

Clinical Presentation

1. Young athletes and adolescents
2. Pain during and after physical activities, especially those demanding vigorous quadriceps contraction

3. Tender, more prominent, edematous, and often warm tibial tuberosity and surrounding area
4. Complete active ROM, but painful passive flexion and resisted extension
5. Compromised quadriceps and hamstrings flexibility
6. Associated biomechanical alterations: valgus knee, pronated foot, and excessive tibial external rotation

Radiographic Evaluation

1. Lateral view with slight internal tibial rotation (using soft-tissue technique) (Fig. 17–7), may show tibial tuberosity fragmentation thick-

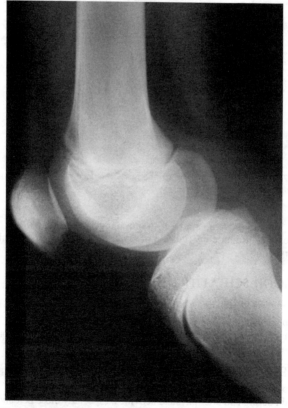

Fig. 17–7. A positive radiograph for Osgood-Schlatter disease.

ened patellar tendon, and dishomogeneous space corresponding to infrapatellar fat pad with obliteration of lower corner

2. Three classes in late stage of disease:
   a. Type 1: Prominent, irregular tibial tuberosity
   b. Type 2: Same as 1 plus small free ossicle located anterosuperior to tuberosity
   c. Type 3: Normal tuberosity with anterosuperior ossicle
3. Ultrasonography can demonstrate other manifestations associated with disease

Treatment

1. Rest from any painful activity to avoid repetitive stresses that can injure ossification nucleus, isolating bony fragments from rest of tuberosity
2. In cases that require strict functional limitations, may need to immobilize joint with femoromalleolar brace for 1–2 wks
3. Control pain with cryotherapy (packages and massages) and NSAIDs
4. Corticosteroid injections and ultrasound therapy not recommended
5. Start functional rehab after acute stage subsides
6. Return to activity when physical examination, radiographs, and sonograms nearly normal, tuberosity nontender, and quadriceps and hamstrings fully recovered
7. Wear padded brace during high-risk sports to protect tuberosity against direct blows

SINDING-LARSEN-JOHANSSON DISEASE

Mechanism of Injury

Traction osteochondritis from functional overload of proximal origin of patellar tendon on lower patellar pole

Clinical Presentation

1. Anterior knee pain ↑ by running activities, going up and down stairs, and kneeling
2. Tenderness of lower patellar pole
3. Pain with resisted knee extension

Radiographic Evaluation

1. Stage 1: Normal appearance
2. Stage 2: Irregular calcifications of lower patellar pole
3. Stage 3: Partial fusion of calcifications
4. Stage 4A: Complete fusion of calcifications, with normal appearance or teardrop shape
5. Stage 4B: Separated ossicle within patellar tendon

Treatment

1. Temporary cessation of all painful activities
2. In acute or severe chronic cases, pain control requires short period of joint immobilization
3. Return to activity after following rehab program similar to that for Osgood-Schlatter disease and when local pain resolves

PES ANSERINUS TENDINITIS

Mechanism of Injury

Insertional tendinitis associated with running, pivoting, jumping, and sudden deceleration, involving tight contraction of inner leg muscles

Clinical Presentation

1. Medial compartment knee pain when running, cutting, or kicking
2. Reproduce pain by palpating tibial insertion area of pes anserinus tendons
3. Passive external rotation and resisted internal rotation during knee flexion-extension also can reproduce pain
4. When associated with symptomatic bursitis, local swelling with crepitation is palpable

Treatment

1. Rest from activity, ice, functional taping, NSAIDs, and hamstring stretching
2. If necessary, infiltrate bursa with corticosteroids
3. Gradual return to activity when pain subsides
4. Orthosis to control external rotation and foot pronation

SEMIMEMBRANOSUS TENDINITIS

Mechanism of Injury

1. Can be 1° lesion from insufficient hamstring flexibility, extensor apparatus malalignment, or training errors
2. Or 2° to intra-articular knee derangements that cause functional overload of musculotendinous unit

Clinical Presentation

1. Posteromedial knee pain during or after long distance running, jumping, repetitive flexion-extension movements, or protracted walking
2. Tenderness localized to posteromedial corner, just below joint line, over tendon, or at tibial insertion
3. With cystic degeneration, local swelling palpable along tendon (pars directa) to tibial insertion

Treatment

1. Rest, ice, NSAIDs, ultrasound, laser, interferential currents, local corticosteroids (if necessary), and hamstring stretching
2. If pain persists, perform bone scintigraphy to rule out medial tibial plateau osteonecrosis
3. Chronic cases that do not respond to conservative therapy may need arthroscopic treatment

ILIOTIBIAL BAND SYNDROME

Mechanism of Injury

1. Overuse syndrome related to repetitive knee flexion-extension movements that cause swelling in structures underlying iliotibial band and band itself
2. Due to friction caused by iliotibial band movement over epicondyle during walking or running
3. Direct blow can provoke syndrome, producing acute hemorrhagic bursitis

Clinical Presentation

1. Lateral knee pain, sometimes radiating toward tibia or over fascia lata
2. Progressive onset of pain, appearing after running or cycling
3. Pain promoted by repetitive knee movements and exacerbated by spring attempts, running with speed, acceleration, etc.
4. Pain resolves immediately upon interruption of training, but returns as soon as running or cycling restarted
5. In advanced cases, pain also present during walking, causing athlete to limp

Physical Examination

1. Tenderness and sometimes crepitus when palpating lateral femoral epicondyle 2–4 cm above joint line and Gerdy's tubercle; no lateral joint line pain
2. No swelling
3. Painless popliteus tendon and lateral collateral ligament
4. In advanced cases, however, whole lateral compartment painful
5. Maneuvers that elicit lateral femoral epicondyle pain confirm diagnosis
   a. Supine athlete performs active knee flexion and extension and examiner maintains compression on focal point; pain greatest at 30–40° flexion
   b. With athlete in lateral decubitus position on uninjured side with hip abducted, pain produced when examiner applies varus stress

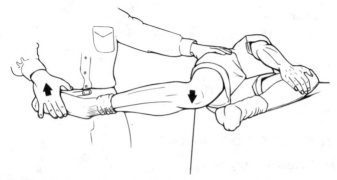

Fig. 17–8. Technique of assessing the flexibility of the iliotibial band (Ober's test). The athlete lies on the uninjured side, and the examiner stabilizes the pelvis with one hand and controls the limb with the other. The hip is first abducted and extended and then adducted toward the table. Tightness of the iliotibial band is demonstrated if the hip remains passively abducted.

   c. Standing on involved leg with knee flexed 30–40° or hopping from knee-flexed position painful

6. Ober's test assesses iliotibial band flexibility (Fig. 17–8).

   a. Patient lies on uninvolved side while examiner stabilizes pelvis with one hand and controls limb with other

   b. First abduct and extend hip and then adduct toward table

   c. Band tightness demonstrated if hip remains passively abducted

7. Negative meniscal and laxity tests

Radiographic Evaluation

1. Negative radiographs

2. Ultrasound may show hypoechoic area (femoral epicondyle) just under iliotibial band

Treatment

1. During acute stage, relative rest for 3–4 days (in severe cases, joint immobilization and no weight bearing)

2. Ice (local application and massages), NSAIDs, ultrasound, microwaves, massage therapy, and laser therapy

3. As soon as possible, stretching exercises for iliotibial band, tensor fascia lata, external rotator muscles of hip, and hamstrings

4. No activity until lateral femoral epicondyle pain disappears; if pain returns, stop activity

5. If conservative therapy fails, surgical intervention necessary

POPLITEUS TENDINITIS

Mechanism of Injury

1. Functional overload of tendon as popliteus muscle checks anterior sliding of femur on tibia and internal tibial rotation
2. Overuse syndrome similar to iliotibial band syndrome seen almost exclusively in endurance runners

Clinical Presentation

1. Unexpected posterolateral knee pain occurs while running downhill or going down stairs
2. Pain with activity can be so severe as to force cessation of activity
3. Immediate symptom relief with brief rest or when running uphill
4. Pain coincides with stance phase of gait when knee flexed 20–30°; reduced by walking with knee fully extended

Physical Examination

1. Lateral compartment tenderness related to popliteus tendon, just anterior or posterior to femoral origin of lateral collateral ligament above joint space
2. Pain over medial tibial margin, above popliteus muscle insertion, and anterior to medial gastrocnemius
3. Maneuvers that elicit pain and help confirm diagnosis:
   a. Resisted internal rotation of leg with knee flexed 90° or fully extended
   b. Resisted knee flexion with leg externally rotated
   c. Passive popliteus muscle stretching with complete external rotation of flexed leg

Treatment

1. Initially, relative rest, ice (locally and massage), NSAIDs, and ultrasound
2. If pain persists, local infiltration of corticosteroids at most painful site (generally femoral origin, but do not place steroid within tendon fibers)
3. Rehab: quadriceps and popliteus stretching and strengthening, hamstring stretching, correction of training errors, and progressive normalization of training to downhill work

BICEPS FEMORIS TENDINITIS

Mechanism of Injury

Overuse injury; traumatic muscle tears more common than pure tendinitis at distal tendon insertion

Clinical Presentation

1. Posterolateral knee pain, progressively aggravated with activity
2. Insidious onset of symptoms
3. Pain to palpation of tendinous insertion to fibular head
4. Resisted active forced knee flexion causes pain

Treatment

1. Initially, rest from activities, ice, NSAIDs, and functional knee taping
2. Rehab: hamstring stretching and strengthening exercises

Extensor Mechanism Problems

EXTENSOR MECHANISM (EM) PROBLEMS

EM Malalignment (EMM)

1. Physical predisposition to patellar problems
2. Predisposition includes bony and muscular abnormalities extending from pelvis to foot
   a. Bony abnormalities (femoral anteversion, genu valgum, and external tibial torsion) can ↑ angle of quadriceps pull
   b. Patella alta, shallow lateral femoral condyle, and patellar shape can affect EM function
   c. Tightness in rectus femoris, iliotibial band, hamstrings, gastrocnemius, soleus, or peripatellar retinaculum may accentuate EM dysfunction
   d. Other factors
      (1) Excessive angular deformities (varus or valgus)
      (2) Functionally short leg
      (3) Knee hyperextension or recurvatum
      (4) Generalized joint laxity
      (5) Abnormal patellar position
      (6) Relative lack of vastus medialis obliquus strength compared to vastus lateralis strength

Classification of EM Problems

1. Primarily instability (patellar dislocation)
2. Mix of instability and pain (patellar subluxation)
3. Pain without instability

ACUTE PATELLAR DISLOCATION

Mechanism of Injury

1. Typically twisting, noncontact mechanism
2. Less often, blow to lateral knee forces knee into valgus
3. Patella completely dislodges from femoral trochlea and rests against lateral femoral condyle

Clinical Presentation

1. Knee collapses, athlete falls
2. Patella remains dislocated until knee fully extended, when patient feels something popping back into place and relief of pain
3. Knee swells shortly after injury
4. Recurrences may follow first acute dislocation, but some patients only experience subluxation

PATELLAR SUBLUXATION

Mechanism of Injury

1. Slipping occurs as athlete attempts to pivot, twist, cut, turn, or otherwise apply rotational stress to knee
2. Patella slips out of normal location briefly, but then spontaneously—and momentarily—reduces

Clinical Presentation

1. No prolonged loss of normal position characteristic of patellar dislocation
2. Some patients with history of subluxation may experience complete dislocation

PAIN SYMPTOMS ONLY

Mechanism of Injury

1. Usually gradual onset of pain syndrome due to overuse
2. Occasionally pain syndrome begins with blunt trauma to anterior knee

Clinical Presentation

1. Pain over anterior knee
   a. Aggravated by activity and prolonged periods of knee flexion
   b. Pain on descending stairs
2. Swelling usually not prominent, but mild puffiness may occur with excessive use of knee.
3. Popping, grinding, or other crepitation around anterior knee
4. Mild, momentary catching episodes with knee extended, so that knee does not seem to bend normally until patella assumes normal position

PHYSICAL EXAMINATION

General Protocol

1. Evaluate patient in upright, sitting, and supine positions
2. While patient stands, walks, and steps up and down from low stool, pay particular attention to action of patellas

Seated Position

1. With knees flexed 90°, note position of patellas
2. Evaluate tibial torsion by viewing knee from above and estimating transmalleolar axis of ankle
3. Assess Q (or tubercle sulcus) angle (Fig. 18–1); residual lateral patellar tendon deviation with knee flexed 90° considered abnormal distal EM alignment
4. Crepitation often palpable in anterior knee when actively extended and flexed
5. As knee extends, patellar tracking should appear as gentle C-shaped curve
6. With patient holding both knees actively flexed at 45°, note muscle forces acting on patellas

Supine Position

1. Assess patellofemoral tenderness and crepitation by compressing patellofemoral joint, both transversely and longitudinally, with knee fully extended and flexed about 30°
2. Evaluate effusion and ROM
3. With knee fully extended and quadriceps tightened, measure Q angle by placing goniometer with pivot point at center of patella
   a. Direct proximal arm toward anterosuperior iliac spine and distal arm along patellar tendon to tibial tuberosity
   b. Q angle ≤10° normal in men; in women, angle may extend to 15°
4. Palpate patellar tendon attachment to inferior patellar pole for tenderness
5. Passively flex and extend knee with fingers over medial patellofemoral region to help find medial synovial plica
6. Assess hip range of motion (especially internal and external rotation); femoral rotational deformities will aggravate patellar problems
7. Evaluate hamstring and heel cord tightness
8. Test patellar instability with knee flexed 20–30°
   a. Apply force along medial patellar edge, displacing it as far laterally as possible (Fig. 18–2)
   b. Hypermobility (compared to opposite knee) is (+) finding

RADIOGRAPHIC EVALUATION

Standard AP and Lateral Views

1. Offer little specific information about patellofemoral joint
2. Rule out other contributing factors (eg, osteoarthritis, osteochondritis dissecans)

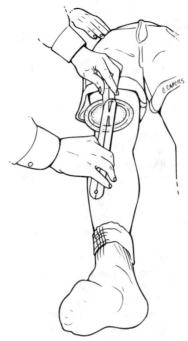

Fig. 18–1. The Q angle can be measured with the patient seated or supine. A goniometer is placed with the pivot point at the center of the patella. The proximal arm is directed toward the anterior superior iliac spine and the distal arm along the patellar tendon to the tibial tuberosity.

Infrapatellar View

1. Useful in evaluating patellofemoral joint disorders; various techniques available
2. Important: obtain radiograph with knee in nearly full extension (Fig. 18-3)
3. Critical points to evaluate
   a. Overall trochlear groove development
   b. Lateral patellar tilting (indicating tightness in lateral supporting structures)
   c. Abnormal lateral patellar displacement out of mid-trochlear groove
   d. Other bony abnormalities: accessory ossification centers along lateral patellar edge, avulsion fracture or calcification along medial edge, or osteochondritis dissecans of patella

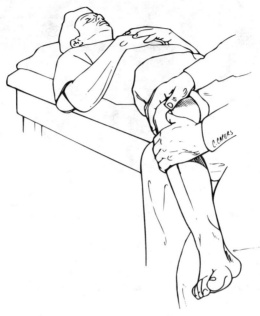

Fig. 18–2. Patellar instability is tested with the patient's knee flexed 20° to 30°. The examiner applies a force along the medial edge of the patella, displacing it as far laterally as possible. Hypermobility compared with the opposite knee is a (+) finding.

Other Imaging Modalities

1. CT: visualizes patellofemoral joint with knee fully extended to diagnose abnormal alignment
2. MRI: assesses articular surface and gives more dynamic picture of patellofemoral tracking
3. Bone scan: shows metabolic component of patellofemoral disease

Arthroscopic Evaluation

1. Performed only when conservative treatment fails and disability warrants surgical intervention
2. Allows full assessment of patellofemoral area
3. Best approach: proximal portal
4. Visible disorders: chondromalacia of patella or trochlea, large medial or suprapatellar plica, excessive lateral patellar tilt, unusual lateral displacement in full extension

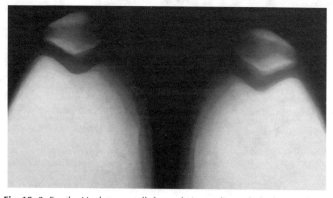

Fig. 18–3. For the Hughston patellofemoral view radiograph the knee is flexed less than 90°. This view, as opposed to the view with the knee flexed, does not show the patella forced to the more distal part of the femoral trochlea.

5. Assess patellar tracking by passively flexing knee; with normal patellar alignment, medial patellar facet contacts medial trochlea by 40° of flexion

TREATMENT

Nonsurgical Treatment

1. Therapeutic Exercises
   a. Control patellar tracking through quadriceps muscle activity by selectively strengthening VMO
   b. Hamstring and gastrocsoleus flexibility
   c. Quadriceps flexibility and iliotibial band stretching
   d. Agility and coordination exercises
   e. Finally, progressive running program returns athlete to activity
2. Adjunctive Therapy
   a. NSAIDs beneficial during therapeutic exercises
   b. Phonophoresis to inflamed area using ultrasound and 10% hydrocortisone cream, especially with patellar tendinitis
   c. Avoid corticosteroid injections because of risk of tendon rupture
   d. Brace or tape for external support
   e. Orthotics for athletes with pronated feet
   f. Avoid prolonged immobilization; even for acute instability, limit immobilization

Surgical Treatment

1. Indicated for significant functional disability despite thorough non-surgical treatment
2. Arthroscopic surgery can be used to debride articular surface chondromalacia, remove loose bodies, or debride hypertrophic infrapatellar fat pad
3. Perform partial synovectomy to remove significantly thickened and fibrotic synovial plica
4. Reserve lateral retinacular release for those with pure pain syndrome rather than patellar instability
5. Direct open surgical repair extremely limited
6. Open EM reconstruction techniques alter muscle forces on patella and change patellar position
7. After arthroscopic or open surgery, appropriate rehab necessary

Meniscal and Chondral Injuries

FUNCTIONAL ANATOMY OF THE MENISCI

Meniscal Movement (Fig. 19–1)

1. Minimal motion of medial meniscus
2. Anteroposterior excursion (ie, extent of movement) of lateral meniscus up to 11 mm

Functional Roles

1. Mechanical spacers contribute to knee joint stability
2. Maintain proper position of femur relative to tibia, thus allowing congruent joint articulation
3. Assist cruciate ligaments in maintaining anteroposterior stability
4. Limit extremes of flexion and extension
5. Aid in joint lubrication

Mechanism of Injury of Meniscal Tears

1. Acute event or degenerative process
2. Noncontact trauma, involving hyperflexion, hyperextension, or rotational (pivoting) forces
3. Twisting or cutting maneuvers that catch meniscus between femoral condyle and tibial plateau may cause tear if forces exceed cartilage's ultimate shear strength

CLASSIFICATION

Based on direction of tear (Fig. 19–2)

Bucket-Handle Tear

1. Most common type of vertical longitudinal tear
2. Most dramatic history and classic signs
3. Can be displaced into intercondylar notch, but once reduced, symptoms may resolve until fragment redisplaces

Vertical Tear

1. Posterior two-thirds meniscus
2. Symptoms when knee extended from flexed position

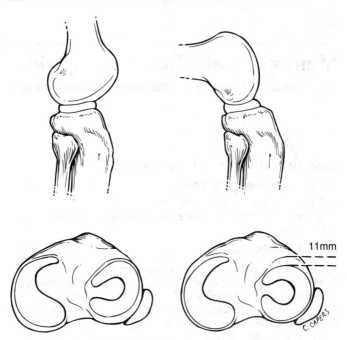

Fig. 19–1. The fact that the horns of the medial meniscus are attached further apart than the horns of the lateral meniscus, that it is firmly anchored by the medial capsular ligaments, and that the medial tibial plateau is more concave, all contribute to the medial meniscus' being relatively constrained. In contrast, the lateral meniscus has an excursion of as much as 11 mm because the horns are attached closer together, there are fewer capsular attachments, and the lateral tibial plateau is flatter.

Transverse (Radial) Tear

1. More common in lateral meniscus and often occurs with other tears
2. Usually at junction of posterior and middle thirds or at posterior horn attachments

Horizontal Tear

1. Frequently in middle third of meniscus
2. Classic symptoms from displacement of unstable portion of meniscus into joint space

Oblique (Flap or Parrot-Beak) Tear

1. Most frequent injury
2. Usually at junction of middle and posterior thirds of medial meniscus

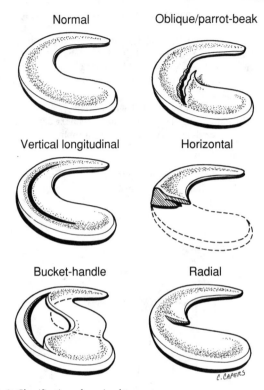

Fig. 19–2. Classification of meniscal tears.

3. Causes catching and popping as athlete pivots or squats and torn meniscus displaces into joint

Degenerative Tear

1. Insidious pain and recurrent effusions
2. Mechanical symptoms (popping, catching, or giving way) depend on severity of tear

Clinical Presentation

1. Symptoms caused by mechanical dysfunction or synovial irritation
2. Hearing or feeling ''pop'' or ''snap'' with pain referred to joint line
3. ↑ pain with rotatory or flexion movements (kneeling, squatting, or pivoting on affected knee)

4. Pain getting into or out of car or difficulty participating in strenuous activity
5. Feeling of insecurity or weakness about knee and giving way
6. Joint locking (loss of terminal 20–30° extension) at injury or as tear extends and gets trapped within joint
7. Locking from chronic tear more subtle and may cause only 5° loss of extension.
8. Sensation of something unusual within joint
9. Joint effusion evolves hours after injury or next day
10. In injuries older than 2 wks, quadriceps atrophy

Physical Examination

1. One of most reliable signs of meniscal injury: joint line pain
2. Anteromedial or anterolateral joint line discomfort with full passive extension suggests meniscal lesion

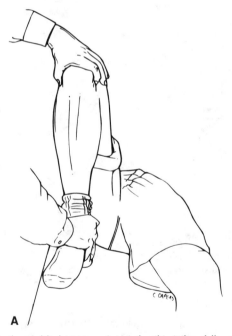

A

Fig. 19–3. In the modified McMurray's test, the tibia is forcefully rotated externally or internally whereas a valgus or varus stress is applied to the knee (depending on which side of the knee is being tested). The knee is started in a flexed position (A) and is moved to an extended position.

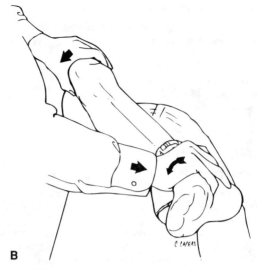

B

Fig. 19–3. (B) While the examiner feels for a pop or clunk at the joint line.

3. Manipulative tests localize pain to joint line or produce clicking due to abnormal meniscal mechanics
   a. McMurray's maneuver more often positive with large flap or bucket-handle tears, but must be correlated with other positive findings
   b. Modified McMurray's test (Fig. 19–3)
      (1) Move flexed knee into extension
      (2) Forcefully rotate tibia externally and internally, applying valgus or varus stress
      (3) (+) test: painful pop or clunk at joint line
   c. Other manipulative tests: Apley's, Steinmann's, and Anderson's
   d. Pain with full flexion, with or without rotation, suggests posterior horn lesion

RADIOGRAPHIC EVALUATION

Plain Radiographs

1. Essential in initial workup of suspected meniscal tear and helpful in ruling out other lesions that may mimic tear
2. With degenerative tears: joint space narrowing, femoral condyle flattening, subchondral bone sclerosis, or osteophyte formation

Double-Contrast Arthrography

Accurate means of diagnosing medial meniscus disease; less accurate for lateral meniscus disorders

MRI

1. Reserved for cases with equivocal findings on physical examination and after failure of conservative treatment
2. More useful in distinguishing medial meniscus tears than lateral meniscus tears

TREATMENT OF MENISCAL TEARS

Conservative Treatment

1. Attempt in all but most severe cases: only locked knee secondary to irreducible, displaced bucket-handle tear requires immediate surgical intervention
2. Treat degenerative tears conservatively unless significant mechanical symptoms unresponsive to conservative therapy develop
3. Use NSAIDs for significant swelling or joint effusion
4. Early Goals
   a. Minimize effusion, normalize gait, pain-free ROM, retard quadriceps atrophy, and maintain cardiovascular endurance
   b. Allow knee to adapt to change in load-bearing capabilities and give sufficient time for tissue healing
5. Intermediate Phase
   a. Improve quadriceps strength and endurance, balance, and proprioception
   b. Swelling and pain dictate pace
6. For optimal results, take knee through progressive activities, including impact-loading and functional exercises specific to individual sport's demands

Surgical Intervention

1. For locked knee secondary to irreducible, displaced bucket-handle tear, perform arthroscopy and partial meniscectomy or meniscal repair to allow ambulation and limit further meniscus or joint surface injury
2. For degenerative tears that cause significant mechanical symptoms despite conservative therapy, arthroscopic debridement of frayed and torn meniscus helpful
3. Partial Meniscectomy: Treatment of choice for most meniscal tears in which pain and swelling persist or significant mechanical symptoms develop despite conservative therapy, and athlete unable to resume activity
4. Meniscal Repair

a. Recommended for tears in vascular region (outer 10–30% of meniscus), longer than 1cm but shorter than 4cm, and unstable on arthroscopic probing

b. Whether arthroscopic or open, repair offers best chance of restoring nearly normal knee kinematics and preventing degenerative arthritis

CHONDRAL LESIONS

Chondromalacia

Cartilage changes of softening and mild arthritis, with fibrillation and surface irregularities

1. Mechanisms of Injury
   a. Acute trauma secondary to direct patellar trauma
   b. Chronic, repetitive, cumulative trauma from alterations in functional conditions or mechanical malalignment (degenerative changes more common in mechanically deranged knees)
   c. Nontraumatic chondromalacia can be associated with nutritional disorders and inborn errors of metabolism

2. Classification
   a. Stage I: Spongy cartilage that on superficial inspection appears normal and feels soft
   b. Stage II: Blister formation
   c. Stage III: Ulceration and fragmentation (Fig. 19–4) with "crab meat" appearance

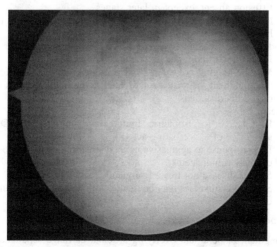

Fig. 19–4. Arthroscopic appearance of Stage III chondromalacia patellae.

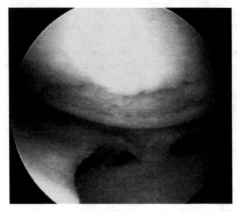

Fig. 19–5. Arthroscopic appearance of Stage IV chondromalacia femoral condyle.

   d. Stage IV: Crater formation and eburnation (Fig. 19–5); with progression, cartilage pieces break off and complete loss of articular cartilage can occur; exposed bone creates crater surrounded by rim of frayed cartilage
3. Clinical Presentation
   a. Mild quadriceps atrophy, joint line tenderness near affected area, pain with McMurray's test, and pain with knee hyperflexion and hyperextension
   b. Effusion absent, except in later stages
   c. No instability, except when chronic ligament instability is underlying cause of chondral problem
4. Radiographic Evaluation
   a. Plain films usually negative and nondiagnostic
   b. May be helpful, however, in identifying axial or patellofemoral malalignment, or unsuspected cause of problem, such as osteochondritis dissecans
5. Treatment
   a. Rest, heat or ice, isometric strengthening program, NSAIDs, and avoidance of exacerbating activities
   b. If no response to aggressive conservative treatment, arthroscopic evaluation indicated
   c. Stage I disease not treated surgically
   d. Stage II-IV diseases may be treated with debridement of unstable cartilage

Osteochondritis Dissecans

   Segment of bone and overlying articular cartilage separated from underlying vascularized bone

1. Mechanism of Injury
   a. Exact cause unknown
   b. May be trauma, nonunion of osteochondral or subchondral fracture, ischemia, or anterior tibial spine impingement against lateral aspect of medial femoral condyle during last few degrees of extension
2. Clinical Presentation
   a. Vague, intermittent, and nonspecific symptoms
   b. Recurrent swelling, irritability, locking, and giving way
   c. Localized tenderness over affected area
   d. Effusion (but may be absent)
   e. Palpable loose body
   f. Quadriceps atrophy, crepitation, and restriction of knee motion
   g. Wilson's sign: pain with knee extension and hip internal rotation; may be specific for osteochondritis dissecans
3. Radiographic Evaluation
   a. Plain radiographs
      (1) Well-circumscribed fragment of subchondral bone separated from femoral condyle and of different density (Fig. 19–6A)
      (2) As fragment separates, may see crater (Fig. 19–6B)
   b. Bone scan, tomography, CT, and MRI may be helpful
4. Arthroscopic Evaluation: helpful for diagnostic confirmation and staging of lesions and in treatment
5. Treatment
   a. Juvenile osteochondritis dissecans
      (1) Conservative treatment effective in treating minimally symptomatic cases
         (a) Minimize immobilization and reserve for acute episodes
         (b) Cast immobilization usually unnecessary; limited-motion hinged knee brace usually sufficient
         (c) Avoiding high-stress activity briefly may relieve symptoms
         (d) Return to activity when evidence of healing
      (2) Perform arthroscopic evaluation if symptoms do not subside within 8–10 wks and bone scan or MRI shows no healing
      (3) Surgical treatments: drilling of intact fragment, pin or screw fixation, bone grafting, and excision of unstable fragment; cautious return to full activity after surgery
   b. Adult-onset osteochondritis dissecans
      (1) Treat conservatively with restriction of athletic activity
      (2) If symptoms persist, perform arthroscopic evaluation
      (3) Stable fragments may be left alone or drilled through articular surface; internal fixation usually not required
      (4) Remove fragments that have been separated from crater longer than few wks

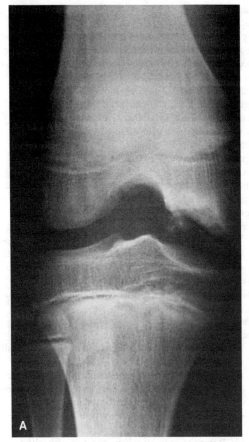

Fig. 19–6A. A well-circumscribed fragment of subchondral bone can be seen separated from the medial femoral condyle.

Chondral Fractures

1. Mechanism of Injury
   a. Direct impact against soft tissue overlying articular surface; fracture line occurs at tide mark, weak zone between calcified and uncalcified cartilage layers
   b. Most common sites: lateral femoral condyle and medial patellar surface
   c. Most often, injury occurs when knee flexed

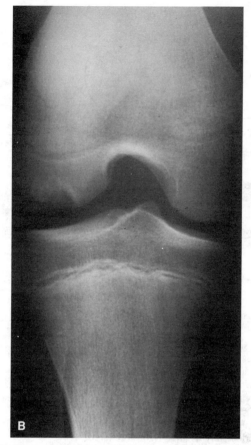

Fig. 19-6B. The crater seen on the lateral femoral condyle indicates osteochondritis dissecans.

2. Classification (Based on Arthroscopic Appearance) (Fig. 19-7)
   a. Traumatic in origin
      (1) Type I: linear crack
      (2) Type II: stellate fracture
      (3) Type III: chondral flap
      (4) Type IV: chondral crater
   b. Degenerative
      (1) Type V: fibrillar appearance
      (2) Type VI: degraded appearance

Type I   Type II   Type III

Type IV   Type V   Type VI

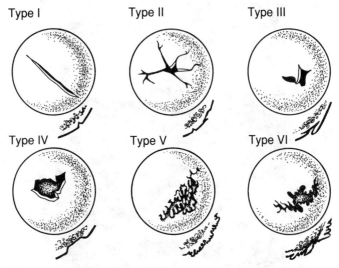

Fig. 19–7. Classification of chondral lesions.

   c. Stellate fractures most common, with flap or crater lesions next most common.
   d. Lesions usually bordered by normal-looking articular cartilage
3. Clinical Presentation
   a. Trauma occurred recently or several months earlier
   b. Symptoms may mimic meniscal problems (eg, locking, catching, giving way).
   c. Chronically painful joint
   d. Often some morning stiffness and impaired ambulation, either periodically or after vigorous exercise
   e. Difficulty with stairs, particularly when ascending
   f. Popping with flexion and extension of knee
4. Physical Examination
   a. Findings suggest meniscus involvement
   b. Few acute, nonspecific findings
     (1) Mild quadriceps atrophy
     (2) Large, small, or absent synovial effusion
     (3) Hemarthrosis uncommon
     (4) Joint line tenderness near chondral lesion
     (5) Painful hyperflexion and hyperextension
     (6) Tenderness directly over femoral condyle or pain with patello-femoral pressure
     (7) No instability unless lesion associated with ligament injury

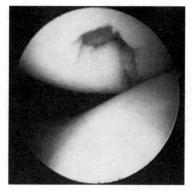

Fig. 19–8. Arthroscopic photograph of a chondral lesion.

    c. Joint aspiration in the acute phase
      (1) Bloody aspirate: possible osteoarticular damage with bleeding
         from subchondral bone
      (2) Hemarthrosis: tear of ACL or other ligament, synovium, or
         peripheral meniscus
      (3) Fat in hemarthrosis: acute osteoarticular fracture
      (4) Synovial fluid white cell count distinguishes post-traumatic
         condition from inflammatory disease
5. Radiographic Evaluation
    a. Pure chondral injuries not seen on standard films and not well
       visualized with arthrography
    b. Bone scan often helpful in showing focal area of joint damage
    c. MRI may also help
6. Arthroscopic Evaluation
    a. Most definitive method of diagnosing chondral fractures
    b. Acute fracture appears as gouged-out defect, flap, or stellate pat-
       tern, depending on mechanism of injury (Fig. 19–8)
7. Treatment
    a. Conservative treatment and 6–8 wks to allow effusion to resolve;
       persistent effusion indicates chondral or meniscus lesion
    b. Surgical treatment of most lesions needed
    c. Goals: to preserve function, restore function, and alleviate pain
    d. Although surgery frequently produces improvement, restoration
       to preinjury condition unlikely
    e. Return to athletic activity may limit longterm improvement

Osteochondral Fractures

1. Mechanism of Injury
    a. Often indirect force, either twisting valgus or varus injury on

straight or slightly flexed knee, or patellar dislocation or subluxation

b. Occasionally, direct force
c. Fracture through articular cartilage involves attached piece of underlying subchondral bone
d. Fracture may or may not be displaced
e. Most common sites: patella, lateral and medial femoral condyles

2. Classification
   a. Exogenous fractures: direct trauma applied to articular cartilage
   b. Endogenous fractures: rotatory and compressive forces applied within knee, and possibly outside trauma

3. Clinical Presentation
   a. Younger athletes
   b. Sudden pain and snap in knee
   c. Chronic symptoms similar to those of meniscus tears

4. Radiographic Evaluation
   a. Standard radiographs useful in demonstrating osteochondral fractures.
      (1) May need multiple views to show fracture and site of origin
      (2) Fragment often appears as very thin line (shell of subchondral bone)
      (3) Sometimes fracture visible only when viewed end-on
      (4) Patellar fractures best seen on sunrise or Merchant views
   b. Osteochondral fractures easily overlooked on MRI

5. Arthroscopic Evaluation: Best means of determining lesion depth and extent

6. Treatment
   a. Treat acute, nondisplaced lesions conservatively with immobilization and avoidance of athletic activity
   b. Treat displaced fractures surgically

Intra-Articular Knee Ligament (Anterior and Posterior Cruciate) Injuries

ACUTE ANTERIOR CRUCIATE LIGAMENT (ACL) INJURIES

Mechanism of Injury

1. Deceleration on planted foot, as in coming down from rebound in basketball or cutting while running
2. Various movements in snow skiing (Fig. 20–1)
   a. Combined external rotation and valgus force, with resultant combined ACL-MCL injury (Fig. 20–1A)
   b. Anteriorly directed force to tibia from back of rigid boot (Fig. 20–1B)
   c. Internal rotation force with knee flexed, resulting in ACL disruption (Fig. 20–1C)
3. ACL and other ligamentous structures can be torn in hyperextension injury
4. Most ACL injuries noncontact, but can involve contact (blow to lateral knee while foot planted)

Clinical Presentation

1. Sound or feel of "pop" at time of injury and inability to continue participation
2. Swelling due to hemarthrosis (within several hrs)

Physical Examination

1. Compare affected knee with contralateral knee
2. Assess effusion and range of motion
3. Lachman's Test (Fig. 20–2)
   a. Most reliable test for ACL tear
   b. Both amount of anterior tibial translation and presence or absence of end point important
4. Other tests: Anterior Drawer Test for anteromedial rotatory instability (AMRI) and Pivot Shift Test

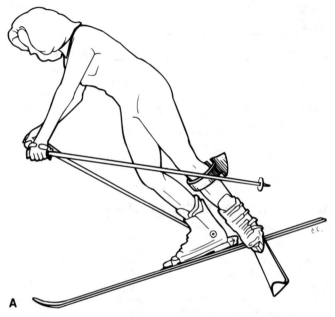

Fig. 20–1. Mechanisms of anterior cruciate ligament (ACL) injury in skiers. (A) The skier falls forward while catching the inside edge of a ski, which produces external rotation and valgus stress, injuring the medial collateral and anterior cruciate ligaments.

5. Instrumented ligament testing (eg, KT-1000) allows objective quantification of tibial translation
6. Evaluate associated injuries, which can significantly ↑ functional instability and future degeneration

Radiographic Evaluation

1. AP, lateral, tunnel, and patellar views rule out associated bone injuries
2. Lateral Capsular Sign (Segond's Fracture) (Fig. 20–3)
   a. Small avulsion fragment from proximal tibial insertion of capsule seen on AP view
   b. Indicates ACL tear and associated lateral ligamentous and capsular injuries
3. MRI (Fig. 20–4)
   a. Not needed for diagnosis of ACL tear, but can assess associated injuries
   b. Age and activity level important factors: young, active patients

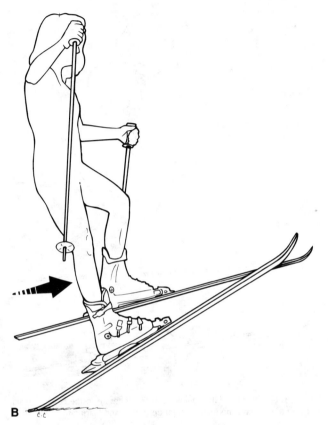

Fig. 20–1. (B) The skier comes down from a jump and lands while leaning backward. The tail of the ski hits first, causing the ski to snap down and resulting in an anterior force to the tibia through the rigid boot.

   involved in aggressive agility sports at higher risk for reinjury with nonsurgical treatment; surgery recommended for those wanting to try to maintain active lifestyle
  c. Patients unwilling or unable to participate in postoperative rehab not good surgical candidates
2. Nonsurgical (Conservative) Management
  a. Treat associated lesions (eg, meniscal tears), manage acute injury, rehab, and establish goals for return to activities
  b. Acute phase

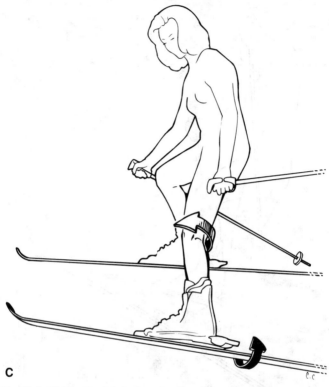

Fig. 20–1. (C) The skier falls backward and catches an inside edge. The ski quickly turns in, causing internal rotation injury, and tearing the ACL.

(1) Manage effusion, regain ROM and muscle control, and restore normal gait pattern
(2) Ice knee on field at time of injury to minimize bleeding and swelling
(3) Perform physical examination (eg, Lachman's test) before hemarthrosis and protective guarding develop
(4) Use knee immobilizer, but not full time or long term
(5) Apply ice frequently to ↓ effusion
(6) Regain normal ROM over several wks with appropriate flexion and extension exercises and patellar mobilization exercises
(7) Perform strengthening exercises to re-establish muscle control and initiate hamstring-dominant gait

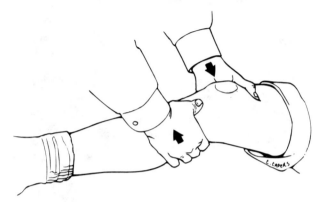

Fig. 20–2. Lachman's test, the most reliable one for an anterior cruciate ligament tear, should be performed with the patient as relaxed as possible, and findings should be compared with those from the opposite limb.

    c. Functional rehab phase
      (1) Starts when full extension and flexion near normal, effusion resolved, hamstring strength $\geq$ 90% of normal, and quadriceps strength > 70% of normal
      (2) Fit patient with brace
      (3) Initiate interval running program, beginning with straight-ahead jogging, progressing to increasing speed, and finally to agility exercises
      (4) Use balancing drills to improve proprioception
      (5) Add sport-specific drills and continue strengthening exercises
    d. Return to activity
      (1) Allow when functional rehab successfully completed
      (2) Based on overall functional assessment of strength, endurance, and agility
      (3) Discourage return to high-risk sports (eg, basketball, football, soccer) because risk of reinjury with meniscal or articular surface damage significant
3. Surgical Management
    a. Timing of surgery
      (1) Delaying surgery 3 or more wks after injury allows acute phase to resolve and ROM to be regained and $\downarrow$ risk of arthrofibrosis
      (2) Earlier surgical intervention needed if multiple ligamentous injuries present
      (3) If extension block present, cause of block and ACL reconstruction can be addressed at same time, or ACL reconstruc-

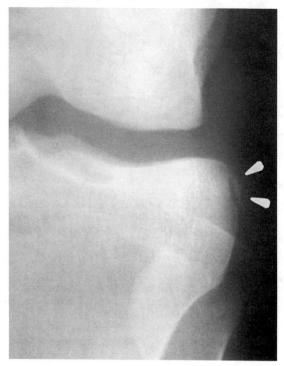

Fig. 20–3. Lateral capsular sign (Segond's fracture). Note the small bony fragment from the lateral tibia, just distal to the joint line. This represents tearing of the tibial insertion of the lateral capsule.

tion can be performed after block has been addressed and extension regained
  b. Evaluation and management of coexisting injuries: perform diagnostic arthroscopy to assess for other injuries (eg, meniscal tears, articular surface damage, osteochondral fractures) and then treat accordingly
  c. Repair or reconstruction options
   (1) Primary ACL repair seldom performed because of high associated failure rate
   (2) Primary repair with augmentation viable, but has several disadvantages
   (3) Primary reconstruction with autograft (usually central third patellar tendon) placed in anatomic position: our treatment of choice

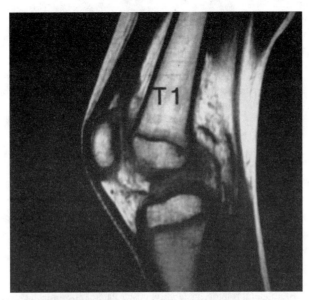

Fig. 20–4. MR image of an acute anterior cruciate ligament tear. Note increased signal intensity in the subchondral area of the lateral femoral condyle and the lateral tibial plateau. The significance of these "bone bruises" remains unclear.

4. Partial ACL Tears
   a. Treat nonsurgically if
      (1) Tear involves < 50% of ligament
      (2) Increased excursion on Lachman's test < 4 mm with good end point
      (3) Pivot shift test negative or trace
   b. Treat surgically if
      (1) Tear involves > 50% of ligament
      (2) Increased excursion on Lachman's test > 4 mm
      (3) Pivot shift test positive

Postoperative Rehabilitation

1. Immediately after surgery, place knee in brace locked in full extension
2. Re-establish ROM and motor control of quadriceps and hamstrings as soon as possible
3. Progress strengthening exercises as in nonsurgical protocol
4. Progression to functional rehab depends on restoration of ROM, adequate muscle control and strength, and resolution of effusion

Return to Activity

1. Predicated on adequate strength and successful completion of functional rehab, including specific drills for sport
2. Average time for return to activity: 9 mos
3. Functional ACL brace (resists varus and valgus loads and hyperextension) recommended for 1st yr after surgery to provide protection from contact-induced reinjury, especially lateral blow

CHRONIC ACL INJURIES

Mechanism of Injury: Present for 6 wks or more, by which time cannot be managed by primary repair

Clinical Presentation

1. ''Giving way'' episodes and general feeling of knee instability
2. At least anteromedial and anterolateral components and maybe posterolateral component

Physical Examination

1. Anteromedial instability: anterior drawer test
2. Anterolateral instability: pivot shift test
3. Posterolateral rotatory instability: posterolateral drawer test, external rotation recurvatum test, and adduction stress test at 30°

Treatment

1. Nonsurgical Management
   a. May be appropriate for older, more sedentary patients with milder instability
   b. Many patients respond well to nonsurgical treatment
   c. Goals: to restore full ROM and strength of extremity (achieving satisfactory muscle strength more difficult with chronic injury if atrophy present)
   d. If functional instability eliminated with rehab, minimal operative intervention may be required
      (1) Arthroscopy for persistent mechanical symptoms (eg, locking or catching), persistent joint line pain, or effusion
      (2) Partial meniscectomy, meniscal repair, synovectomy, or ACL stump debridement may assist overall rehab and obviate surgical stabilization
2. Surgical Management
   a. Selection criteria similar to those for acute ACL injury
      (1) Also important: 2° instability, muscle atrophy, and arthritic changes
      (2) Symptomatic functional instability with repeated effusions and giving way, despite bracing and adequate trial of rehab, requires surgical stabilization

b. Extra-articular reconstruction
   (1) For anteromedial instability, surgery aimed at posterior oblique ligament reconstruction
   (2) For anterolateral instability, surgery aimed at reconstructing lateral middle third capsule and iliotibial tract and transferring long head of biceps tendon into reconstructed tract
   (3) For posterolateral rotatory instability, posterolateral reconstruction should only be done if
      (a) External rotation recurvatum (+)
      (b) Posterolateral drawer test > 1 +
      (c) Lateral meniscus absent and opening = 2 to 3 mm with adduction stress
c. Intra-articular reconstruction
   (1) For active patients with chronic functional instability, especially with 2° instability, degenerative changes, or meniscal damage
   (2) Autografts
      (a) Most popular technique: autogenous bone-patellar tendon-bone graft using central third patellar tendon with bone plugs from interior patellar pole and tibial tubercle
      (b) Advantages: ligament strength, strong fixation with early plug consolidation, and no disease transmission
      (c) Disadvantages: donor site morbidity (eg, patellofemoral joint pain), mechanical problems, and ↑ operative time
   (3) Allografts
      (a) Cadaver allograft placement and bone plug fixation as for autografts
      (b) ACL allografts provide functional replacement for ACL-deficient knees
      (c) Advantages: ↓ early morbidity and patellofemoral trauma, ↓ operative time, minimal surgical incisions, and possible ↓ time to functional return
      (d) Disadvantages: possibility of disease transmission and ↑ time for revascularization requires ↑ period of protection

ACUTE POSTERIOR CRUCIATE LIGAMENT (PCL) INJURIES

1. Most common cause: anteroposterior blow to tibia with knee flexed
2. ''Isolated'' or interstitial tear: athlete falls on flexed knee while foot is plantar flexed (Fig. 20–5)
3. Isolated tear can also occur with forced knee hyperflexion while foot dorsiflexed
4. Unexpected, sudden knee hyperextension can cause injury; if knee forced into 30° extension, posterior capsule tears first, then PCL, and usually ACL also

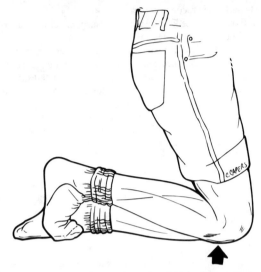

Fig. 20–5. The mechanism of injury for an interstitial or isolated tear of the PCL can be a fall on the flexed knee with the foot in plantar flexion.

5. Rotational forces with associated valgus or varus stress may also cause PCL tears, medial or lateral collateral ligament tears, and possibly ACL tears

Clinical Presentation

1. Minimal swelling with mild bloody effusion: swelling within 2 hrs and less tense than that seen with ACL injuries or patellar dislocation
2. Posterior knee tenderness in popliteal fossa or posterolateral corner
3. Abrasion, anterior aspect of proximal tibia
4. Walking with knee flexed to avoid painful extension
5. Peroneal nerve damage from varus force that injures posterolateral ligaments

Physical Examination

1. Stability tests based on posterior translation of tibia in relation to femur
2. Sag Test (Fig. 20–6)
   a. Flex both knee and hip to 90°
   b. Tibial tubercle "disappears" or "drops back" on lateral inspection of affected knee compared with normal knee
   c. If PCL ruptured, gravity causes posterior displacement of tibia in relation to femur

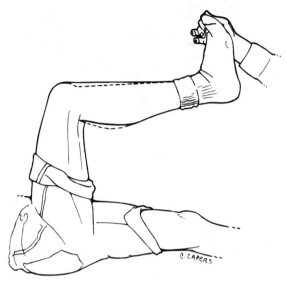

Fig. 20–6. A positive sag test result indicates a ruptured PCL.

3. Posterior Drawer Test (Fig. 20–7)
   a. Posterior drawer sign (posterior force to tibia creates posterior movement) sensitive for PCL injury
   b. If test remains positive with tibia in internal rotation, diagnosis confirmed
4. Other Tests
   a. Quadriceps Active Test: with knee flexed 90°, patient tenses quadriceps and tibia reduced into normal position
   b. Godfrey's Test: with both hip and knee flexed 90°, examiner holds heel and compares posteriorly displaced tibial tubercle with uninjured side
   c. Shelbourne's Dynamic Posterior Shift Test: with hip flexed 90° and heel supported in examiner's hand, slowly and fully extend knee; clunk or jerk felt as knee reduces
   d. Posterior Lachman's Test: done in same flexed position (approximately 30°) as anterior Lachman's test, but posterior end point felt
   e. Reverse Pivot Shift Test: may indicate PCL injury, but best for detecting posterolateral rotatory instability; apply valgus load to flexed knee and then bring knee into extension; reduction occurs when joint brought from subluxated position (flexed) into extension

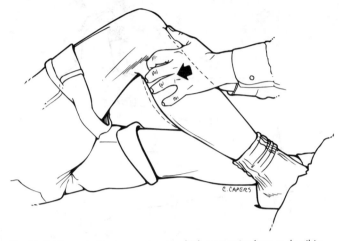

Fig. 20–7. The posterior drawer sign, in which a posterior force to the tibia creates posterior movement, is a sensitive test for PCL injury.

5. Posterolateral drawer test and external rotation recurvatum tests negative with PCL injury, but positive with posterolateral injury

Radiographic Evaluation

1. Lateral view: posterior tibial translation or sag
2. AP stress views help demonstrate injury severity
   a. With isolated tear, tibia moves posteriorly
   b. More than 10 mm displacement indicates associated ligament injuries (ie, posterolateral)
3. Posterior tibial avulsion fractures indicate PCL injury
4. Acute injury causes increased MRI signal intensity in PCL substance (Fig. 20–8)

Treatment

1. Generally, isolated PCL tear is interstitial and treated nonsurgically
2. Treat bony avulsions by surgically reattaching bone fragment with sutures or screws
3. Treat PCL injury associated with other ligament injury surgically; repair coexisting ligament injuries as anatomically as possible in acute phase
4. Augmentation done with any primary PCL repair
   a. Patellar tendon best for augmentation
   b. Limited success with other autograft tissues

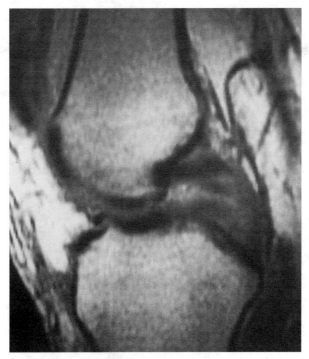

Fig. 20–8. MRI can show disruption of the PCL.

Rehabilitation

1. Early motion desirable
2. Emphasize quadriceps strengthening during first 2 wks after injury
3. During next 4 wks, add hamstring strengthening
4. Return to activity when athlete has regained full ROM, and strength, power, and endurance equal to that in uninjured knee

CHRONIC PCL INJURIES

Mechanism of Injury

1. PCL dynamically supported by quadriceps, with proprioceptive control of knee dependent on intact quadriceps mechanism
2. Increased laxity from PCL injury allows shearing forces to occur in knee; when normal proprioceptive control fails, symptoms become manifest and progress

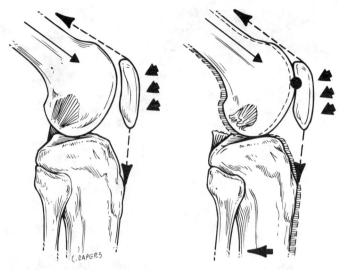

Fig. 20–9. A functioning quadriceps mechanism is necessary for proprioceptive control of the knee. The static stability provided by the cruciate ligament protects the patellofemoral mechanism and the menisci and stops the femur from being driven into the tibia in deceleration and descending movements.

Clinical Presentation

1. Symptoms of instability or laxity: persistent pain, catching, swelling, or recurrent episodes of instability
2. PCL rupture causes difficulties in running downhill, decelerating, stopping after running, and descending stairs
3. Combined PCL and other major ligament injuries usually associated with posterolateral disruption, causing severe subluxations and instability (particularly with hyperextension and varus force)
4. Meniscal tears or articular surface damage contribute to increased incidence of osteoarthritis

Treatment

1. Goal: to correct disability and restore knee function
2. Conservative treatment: rehabilitative exercises and teaching of proprioceptive control mechanisms (Fig. 20–9)
3. Criteria for surgical intervention similar to those of acute PCL injuries.

Extra-Articular Knee Ligament and Capsular Injuries

INJURIES TO THE MEDIAL LIGAMENT COMPLEX (MLC)

Functional Anatomy of the MLC

1. 1° Function: To resist valgus and external rotation forces about knee and, to a lesser degree, anterior tibial translation with tibia in external rotation
2. 2° Function: To protect medial meniscus

Mechanism of Injury

1. Contact Stresses
   a. Cause many MLC disruptions
   b. Acute Anteromedial Rotatory Instability (AMRI): Contact force applied to lateral knee or proximal tibia when foot planted on ground, resulting in valgus and external rotation stress
   c. Disruption of medial capsular ligament and overlying tibial collateral ligament: Pure valgus stress
   d. Disruption of posterior oblique ligament
      (1) Combined valgus stress and external rotation
      (2) As valgus force ↑, tibial collateral ligament and middle third medial capsular ligament also injured, resulting in AMRI
      (3) With further stress, ACL may be disrupted, resulting in anterolateral rotatory instability (ALRI)
2. Noncontact Injuries
   a. MLC can be disrupted by fall or sudden valgus stress (eg, when snow skier ''catches an edge'') or sudden external rotation force (eg, when water ski catches in water or cyclist places foot on ground while moving)
   b. Deceleration, cutting, twisting, and pivoting maneuvers may disrupt MLC
      (1) Depending on stress involved, ACL, medial meniscus, and PCL may also be injured
      (2) Knee dislocation can occur, and with increasing valgus stress, lateral tibial plateau fracture

Classification

1. Grade I MLC Sprain: microtearing of ligament fibers, usually from valgus stress, with interstitial hemorrhage and localized tenderness but no demonstrable instability
2. Grade II MLC Sprain: more ligament fiber involvement and altered ligament integrity, usually due to moderate trauma, with minimal to mild clinical instability
3. Grade III MLC Sprain: complete ligament disruption, usually due to severe trauma, with associated significant clinical instability

Clinical Presentation

1. General
   a. Audible or palpable "pop" may occur at time of injury, but usually associated with ACL injury
   b. With pure MLC injury, less pronounced swelling; even with associated ACL disruption, swelling may be mild because hemarthrosis extravasates into soft tissues
   c. Functional instability can manifest as giving way secondary to reflex quadriceps inhibition from pain and weakness
   d. Muscle splinting and gait alteration may allow walking without giving way
   e. Limited extension (usually associated with meniscal tear) often secondary to muscle spasm and pain as medial ligament structures tighten with increasing extension; "pseudolocking" occurs several hrs after injury
   f. ↓ flexion due to pain from soft-tissue injury
   g. MLC palpation frequently reveals defect in area of ligament disruption
2. Grade I MLC Sprain
   a. Pain localized to medial joint
   b. Patient usually ambulatory, but gait may be antalgic and knee extension limited due to spasm and pain
   c. Localized swelling and tenderness over medial ligaments, but no demonstrable instability
3. Grade II MLC Sprain
   a. Localized swelling over injured structures and tenderness to direct palpation
   b. Patient may be ambulatory, but with limited extension due to spasm and pain
   c. Mild instability
4. Grade III MLC Sprain
   a. Degree of instability depends on ligament structures involved and status of secondary restraints
   b. Pain in immediate postinjury period may be < with Grade I or II sprains

   c. Swelling may represent hemarthrosis
   d. Greater limitation of motion secondary to spasm and pain
   e. Associated injuries more likely

Physical Examination

1. Abduction Stress Test
   a. Most important clinical test for evaluating MLC
   b. Perform at 30° flexion (Fig. 21–1) to evaluate tibial collateral

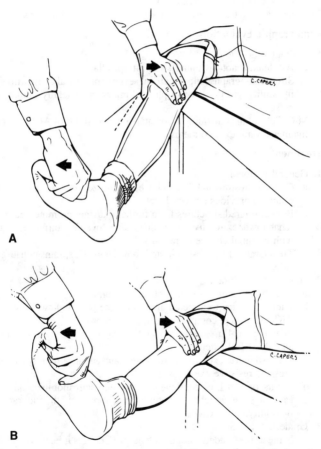

Fig. 21–1. A. The abduction stress test at 30° of knee flexion tests the integrity of the medial ligament complex. B. The abduction stress test at full extension.

      ligament and middle third medial capsular ligament, and in full extension to evaluate PCL and posteromedial capsular structures

  c. Patient supine with thigh supported on table; swing leg gently to side and grasp forefoot with one hand, applying pressure to lateral knee with other hand

  d. Move foot back and forth repeatedly from midline, applying counterpressure laterally at knee

  e. Evaluate abnormal motion and rate from 0–5 mm, 5–10 mm, or > 10 mm pathologic ''opening''

  f. With increasing instability and greater involvement of other structures, end point becomes softer (ie, ''mushy'')

2. Other stability tests: perform to assess for associated injuries

Radiographic Evaluation

1. Radiographic Views
  a. AP, lateral, notch (tunnel), and infrapatellar
  b. Stress radiographs help document severity of medial compartment instability and presence of physeal injury in skeletally immature persons

2. MRI: helpful in confirming associated injuries (status of ACL, lateral ligament complex, and menisci)

Treatment

1. General protocol
  a. Goals: to restore stability to knee, maximize function, and allow return to previous activity level
  b. Protect injured structures from further damage, promote healing, rehab lower extremity, and evaluate knee for safe return to activity with minimal chance of reinjury
  c. Treat Grades I and II sprains and some Grade III sprains nonsurgically

2. Grade I MLC Sprain
  a. Crutch ambulation for protection and comfort
  b. Intermittent ice to affected area to reduce pain and swelling
  c. RICE (rest, ice, compression, and elevation)
  d. Injecting local anesthetic into tender area may alleviate discomfort and allow full extension
  e. Start isometric exercises immediately and advance rapidly to progressive resistive exercises
  f. As discomfort ↓, discontinue crutches and start mobilization
  g. More aggressive rehab structured to restore strength, endurance, flexibility, and ROM

3. Grade II MLC Sprain
  a. Same as for Grade I sprain: crutches, RICE, plus injection of local anesthetic if necessary
  b. Patients usually more comfortable in rehab brace that allows full

motion but offers protection against valgus stress on injured structures

c. Protected weight bearing with crutches

d. Start isometric exercises immediately and advance rapidly to progressive resistive exercises as comfort allows

e. Gently test stability weekly; stability usually maximizes within several wks

f. As discomfort diminishes and stability returns, discontinue crutches and brace and start aggressive rehab

4. Grade III MLC Sprain

a. Place patients with diffusely swollen knees, especially with hemarthrosis and marked limitation of motion, on crutches and program of RICE, brace or splint, and early exercises to reduce pain, swelling and limitation of motion

b. Consider nonsurgical treatment if no associated intra-articular injuries (eg, meniscal or ACL tears)

(1) Prolonged crutch ambulation and limited-motion brace to protect against extremes of motion for 4–6 wks

(2) Gently test stability to monitor progress

c. Grade III sprains with significant instability traditionally treated by primary open surgical repair acutely with good results

(1) Repair associated injuries (eg, meniscal and ACL tears) at same time

(2) Postop, hold lower extremity in limited-motion brace for 6 wks

(3) Traditionally, restrict last 30° extension

(4) Currently, some surgeons treat Grade III sprains with early protected motion from 0–90°, especially when combined with ACL reconstruction

POSTEROLATERAL ROTATORY INSTABILITY (PLRI)

Functional Anatomy

1. Posterolateral knee is complex, interlinked musculotendoligamentous unit known as arcuate complex (Fig. 21–2)

2. Arcuate complex deficit produces greatest dysfunction and potential impairment near complete extension

3. Removing posterolateral restraints ↑ external tibial rotation; magnitude depends on angle of knee flexion

4. Arcuate complex: principal restraint to lateral opening

5. Posterolateral dysfunction can ↑ internal rotation laxity and external rotation

Mechanism of Injury

1. Injury to arcuate complex, not PCL, causes PLRI

a. PLRI is abnormal external rotation and posterior subluxation of lateral tibial plateau in relation to lateral femoral condyle

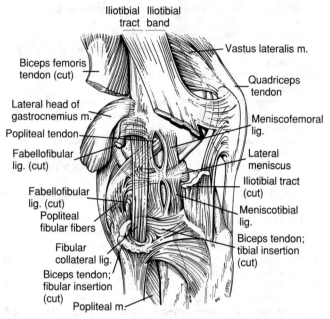

Fig. 21–2. Anatomy of the lateral aspect of the knee, including the arcuate ligament.

    b. Abnormal rotation occurs only with intact PCL

    c. Instability can be isolated or combined with anterolateral or anteromedial instability, or both

2. Typical mechanism of injury: hyperextension and external rotation

3. PLRI can result from contact injury caused by direct blow or noncontact injury caused by indirect force applied to knee

    a. Common in football: direct blow to extended knee, often from anteromedial side → forceful hyperextension and simultaneous external tibial rotation (Fig. 21–3)

    b. Noncontact hyperextension injuries related to sudden or unexpected upper leg and body deceleration, which acts on posterolateral knee structures as lever on fixed or planted foot

4. With knee extended, posterolateral capsule is principal restraint to injury, and concomitant PCL tears rarely seen

5. Combined posterolateral and PCL injuries typically occur from direct anterior blow to flexed knee

Clinical Presentation

1. PLRI and other injuries: athlete cannot bear weight on injured leg and usually seeks medical attention promptly

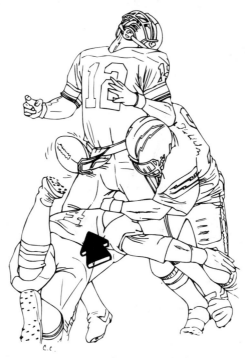

Fig. 21–3. The mechanism of injury for the posterolateral structures is often a direct blow to the extended knee from the anteromedial side, causing forceful hyperextension and simultaneous external tibial rotation.

2. Isolated PLRI: athlete may have little swelling, walk with limp, and not seek medical attention until days or wks after injury

3. Chronic PLRI: most frequent complaint is ''giving way backward'' into hyperextension, causing athlete to unconsciously assume flexed-knee gait; twisting, pivoting, and cutting difficult and athlete unable to ''push off'' with affected leg; pain localized along medial joint line

Physical Examination

1. Posterolateral Drawer Test (Fig. 21–4)
 a. Perform with knee in 90° and 30° flexion
 b. Place both hands on proximal tibia with thumbs on either side of tibial tubercle
 c. Rotate leg and foot externally, and apply repeated push and external rotation motions

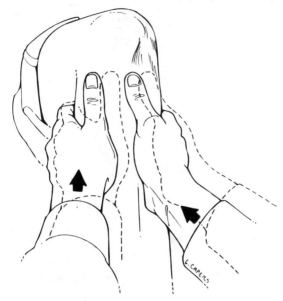

Fig. 21–4. The posterolateral drawer test is used to measure posterior and external rotational translation of the tibia.

    d. Look and feel for posterior and external rotational tibial translation while pushing
    e. Compare results with uninjured knee
2. Posterior Drawer Test
    a. Evaluates PCL integrity
    b. Perform with leg in neutral and internal rotation
    c. Compare with results of posterolateral drawer test
3. If patient has PLRI and intact PCL, posterior drawer sign absent when knee rotated internally
4. External Rotation Recurvatum Test
    a. Demonstrates abnormal motion of femur in relation to tibia with knee extended
    b. Perform with patient supine and leg extended
    c. Place one hand behind knee and with other hand hold medial forefoot and lift lower leg, maximally extending knee (Fig. 21–5)
    d. Visualize and feel (with hand behind knee) external rotation recurvatum
    e. Compare external rotation recurvatum in injured and uninjured knees
5. Physical Signs

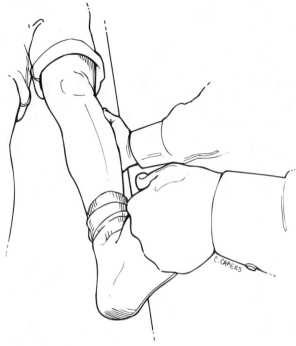

Fig. 21–5. Side-to-side comparison during the external rotation recurvatum test is done by lifting the patient's extremities by the big toe of each foot and watching for external rotation recurvatum in the injured extremity.

   a. Abrasions or ecchymosis on medial knee or upper shin
   b. Peroneal nerve injury, either transient paresthesia or complete palsy

Radiographic Evaluation

1. "Arcuate Sign"
   a. Fragment of bone avulsed from fibular head
   b. In acutely injured knee, indicates posterolateral ligamentous injury
2. MRI
   a. Often useful in determining if ligamentous and osseous injuries of posterolateral knee exist, but not helpful in assessing specific pattern or exact location
   b. Most helpful in assessing integrity and anatomy of cruciate ligaments and menisci

Treatment

1. Acute PLRI
   a. Surgically repair acute ligament or tendon injuries with direct ligament-to-ligament and soft tissue-to-bone suture techniques
   b. With isolated PLRI in which ACL torn (combined PLRI-ALRI), repair capsular and extra-articular injuries first; perform ACL reconstruction when full extension can be included in early rehab
2. Chronic PLRI
   a. For combined PLRI-ALRI in which PLRI severe, perform extra-articular and capsular reconstruction
   b. When less severe subluxation is PLRI, consider combining intra-articular cruciate and extra-articular capsular surgery
   c. 3 general methods of ligament reconstruction for chronic PLRI: arcuate complex advancement and reefing; popliteal bypass; and fibular collateral ligament reconstruction

Traumatic Ankle and Foot Injuries

ANKLE SPRAINS

Lateral Ligament Sprains

1. Mechanism of Injury
   a. Lateral ligaments injured by inversion or varus tilt only when ankle incompletely loaded (eg, during initial contact with ground) and possibly because of internal rotation (Fig. 22–1)
   b. Forced plantar flexion with adduction causes rupture of anterior talofibular ligament (ATFL), followed by partial rupture of calcaneofibular ligament (CFL); with continued force, CFL ruptures completely, followed by posterior talofibular ligament (PTFL)
2. Classification
   a. Grade I: mild sprain
   b. Grade II: moderate sprain
   c. Grade III: severe sprain
3. Clinical Presentation (48 hrs after injury)
   a. Mild sprain: minimal swelling, good ROM, and able to bear weight comfortably without crutches
   b. Moderate sprain: more pronounced swelling, ROM limited to 0–30° flexion, and crutches or cane needed to bear weight on affected extremity
   c. Severe sprain: marked swelling, ecchymosis laterally, minimal pain-free ROM, and unable to bear weight on affected extremity
4. Physical Examination
   a. General Observations
      (1) Diffusely swollen, plantar flexed, ecchymotic, tender ankle
      (2) Tenderness usually at anterolateral ankle and CFL
      (3) Medial ankle and syndesmosis may be tender and swollen
      (4) Delay stability tests until pain and swelling have subsided (4–7 days after injury)
   b. Anterior Drawer Test (Fig. 22–2)
      (1) Mainly assesses ATFL integrity
      (2) Perform with ankle in neutral position and plantar flexed

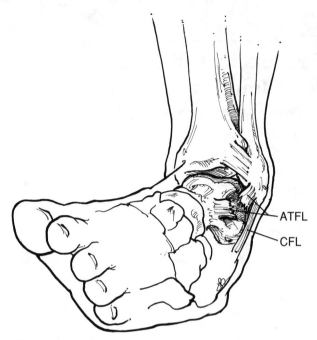

ATFL

CFL

Fig. 22–1. "Inversion" or varus tilt, injury to lateral ankle ligaments.

  (3) Stabilize tibia with 1 hand while other hand directs anterior force to heel
  (4) When ATFL ruptured and anterior force applied to talus, anterolateral talar edge shifts approximately 1 cm forward, out of ankle mortise
 c. Inversion Stress Test (Talar Tilt Test)
  (1) Mainly assesses CFL integrity
  (2) Perform with ankle in neutral position or slight plantar flexion
  (3) Stabilize tibia with 1 hand, while other hand applies varus stress at calcaneocuboid joint
 d. Interpretation of Findings
  (1) Combined ATFL tenderness, lateral hematoma discoloration, and positive anterior drawer test almost always indicate lateral ligament sprain
  (2) Absence of ATFL tenderness excludes ankle ligament rupture
  (3) No hematoma and negative anterior drawer test indicate intact capsular ligament

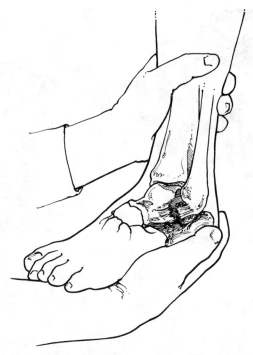

Fig. 22–2. The anterior drawer test demonstrates instability of the ATFL.

5. Radiographic Evaluation
   a. AP and lateral views demonstrate ligament-avulsion fractures and rule out other bony lesions
   b. Stress radiographs can document instability demonstrated during physical examination (Fig. 22–3)
      (1) Talar tilt $\geq 6°$ equals anterior drawer > 3 mm and indicates ligament injury
      (2) Talar tilt $>10°$ with inversion stress test, compared to opposite ankle, represents significant chronic instability
6. Treatment
   a. Treat all initial acute sprains nonsurgically, with early functional mobilization by way of immediate rehab
      (1) Functional treatment: short period of protection (elastic bandage or plaster casting immobilization) followed by early ROM exercises and neuromuscular training

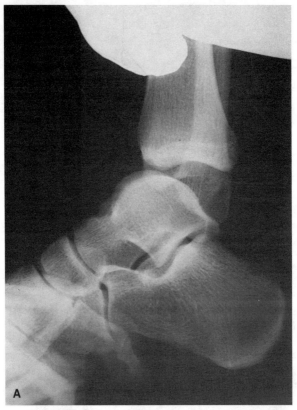

Fig. 22–3. A. Radiograph shows instability of the ATFL. B. Inversion stress test (talar tilt test) demonstrates instability of the CFL.

      (2) Provides quickest recovery of full ROM and return to activity without producing any more mechanical or functional instability than casting alone or surgery

  b. Goals of initial treatment: to minimize pain, swelling, and stiffness

      (1) Avoid casting in favor of elastic bandage or pneumatic compression splint (Fig. 22–4) if possible to prevent muscle atrophy and joint stiffness

      (2) Reserve casting for patients with severe pain and swelling and so much guarding that they will not move ankle at all

      (3) Remove cast after 1 wk, and apply elastic bandage or pneumatic compression splint

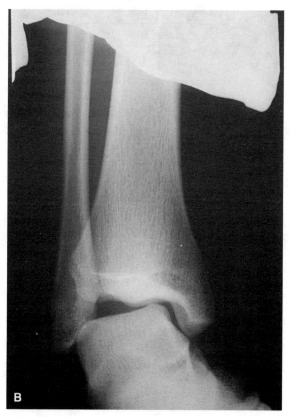

Fig. 22–3. *(continued).*

(4) Start partial weight bearing immediately and dorsiflexion and plantar flexion ROM exercises as tolerated

(5) Rest, elevate, and ice

(6) As soon as possible, start strengthening with isometric exercises, advancing to progressive isotonic and isokinetic resistance exercises

(7) When strength permits, start proprioceptive exercises

(8) After normal strength returns, allow running and agility activities

(9) Emphasize heel cord stretching throughout rehab to prevent recurrent sprains

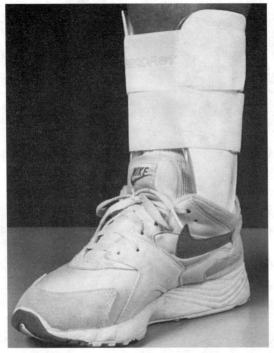

Fig. 22–4. Use of pneumatic compression splint to protect a sprained ankle.

     (10) Elastic bandage or pneumatic splint use
        (a) Several days if swelling minimal
        (b) 6 wks if hematoma obvious or pain severe due to swelling
        (c) Discontinue when athlete feels comfortable and confident
        (d) Continue protection for athletes with recurrent sprains when participating in agility sports
7. Indications for Surgery
   a. Chronic functional instability (giving way) and documented mechanical instability
   b. No benefit from nonsurgical treatment
   c. Young athletes predisposed to lateral ligament injuries who are involved in ball sports
8. Postop Regimen
   a. Immediately postop, apply dorsal splint for 3–5 days

b. After splint removed, initiate prescribed exercises
c. 1 wk postop remove sutures, protect joint with elastic bandage or pneumatic splint for 5 wks, and continue rehab
d. Full weight bearing as tolerated

Syndesmosis Sprains

1. Mechanism of Injury
   a. Often due to eversion-external rotation injury, as when athlete stopped and pushed back on planted foot (Fig. 22–5)
   b. Tibiofibular syndesmosis ligament injuries usually associated with ankle fractures
2. Classification (''frank'' ankle diastasis without fracture)
   a. Type I: straight lateral fibular subluxation
   b. Type II: straight lateral fibular subluxation with plastic deformity of fibula
   c. Type III: posterior rotatory subluxation of fibula
   d. Type IV: superior dislocation of talus
3. Physical Examination
   a. Tenderness over distal tibiofibular and deltoid ligaments
   b. Positive ''squeeze'' test at mid-calf

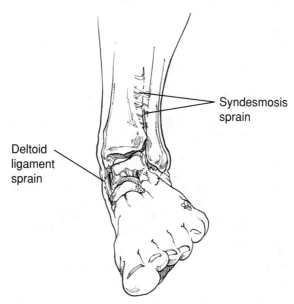

Fig. 22–5. Eversion and external rotation injury resulted in a syndesmosis sprain.

4. Radiographic Evaluation
   a. AP, lateral, and mortise views
   b. Stress views with external rotation may confirm diagnosis
5. Treatment
   a. Depends on severity of injury and degree of instability
   b. If no instability, bear weight as tolerated using elastic bandage or pneumatic splint for protection while progressing through rehab as for inversion sprain
   c. If radiographs normal but laxity on stress testing, immobilize ankle in long-leg cast for 6 wks; obtain follow-up radiographs during first 3 wks
   d. If radiographs show acute syndesmotic disruption or patient develops diastasis during conservative treatment, screw fixation necessary for stabilization
      (1) After wounds heal, apply splint, start ROM exercises, and permit protective weight bearing as tolerated
      (2) Remove screw 8–12 wks after surgery and accelerate rehab
      (3) Return to activity 3–4 mos following surgery

Medial Ligament Sprains

1. Mechanism of Injury
   a. Forced external rotation and abduction (may be combined with forced plantar flexion or neutral position) causes partial rupture of deltoid ligament (Fig. 22–6)
   b. Deltoid ligament tears typically associated with syndesmosis injury or fibular fracture, but can also be injured during lateral ligament sprains; isolated tears of deltoid ligament extremely rare
2. Examination
   a. Tenderness over deltoid ligament and anterior syndesmosis, lateral malleolus, or proximal fibula, depending on other injuries
   b. Evaluate ankle joint stability and posterior tibial tendon function
   c. Routine and stress radiographs assess stability and help determine treatment
3. Treatment
   a. Manage rare, isolated deltoid ligament tear or deltoid ligament injury with stable syndesmosis sprain nonsurgically, with protected mobilization or cast immobilization
   b. Treat unstable syndesmosis rupture surgically; approach deep deltoid ligament surgically only when necessary to extricate it to reduce ankle joint

OTHER TRAUMATIC INJURIES TO THE ANKLE AND HINDFOOT

Ankle Fractures

1. Mechanism of Injury

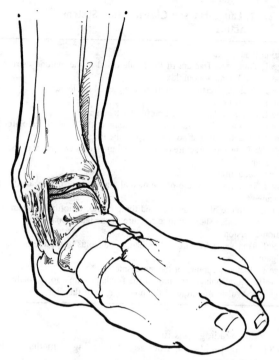

Fig. 22–6. Forced external rotation and abduction injury resulted in partial rupture of the deltoid ligament.

  a. Only those injuries involving ankle mortise disruption considered ankle fractures
  b. Usually due to indirect forces: adduction, abduction, or rotation between lower leg and foot
2. Classification: Based on mechanism of injury, foot position, and direction of force at time of injury (Table 22–1)
3. Clinical Presentation
  a. Audible "pop" at time of injury
  b. Ability to bear weight on affected extremity depends on degree of injury
  c. Joint deformity
  d. Tenderness to knee in certain ankle fractures
4. Radiographic Evaluation
  a. AP, lateral, and mortise (20° internal rotation oblique) views. If pain or tenderness proximal to ankle, obtain 2 views of lower leg

Table 22–1. Lauge-Hansen Classification System for Ankle Fractures

Supination-Adduction
   Stage I: Transverse fracture of the fibula distal to the plafond or rupture of the lateral ligament complex
   Stage II: Includes vertical fracture of the medial malleolus
Supination-Eversion
   Stage I: Injury to the anterior tibiofibular ligament
   Stage II: Spiral-oblique fracture of the fibula at the level of the plafond
   Stage III: Fracture of the posterior lip of the tibia
   Stage IV: Transverse fracture of the medial malleolus or rupture of the deltoid ligament
Pronation-Adduction
   Stage I: Transverse fracture of the medial malleolus or rupture of the deltoid ligament
   Stage II: Rupture of the anterior and the posterior tibiofibular ligaments
   Stage III: Includes short oblique fracture of the lateral malleolus
Pronation-Eversion
   Stage I: Transverse fracture of the medial malleolus or rupture of the deltoid ligament
   Stage II: Includes rupture of the syndesmosis
   Stage III: Spiral-oblique fracture of the fibula proximal to the plafond
   Stage IV: Avulsion fracture of the posterior lip of the tibia

   b. Evaluate radiographs for
      (1) Medial malleolar fracture, or widening of medial malleolus-talus space
      (2) Fibular fracture, its relationship to tibial plafond (ie, at, above, or below), and orientation (eg, transverse, oblique, comminuted)
      (3) Distal tibiofibular joint displacement to assess syndesmosis competence
      (4) Talar displacement from normal anatomic position beneath tibia
5. Treatment
   a. Treat ankle fractures with or without internal fixation; final results depend on accuracy and maintenance of reduction
   b. Manage isolated, nondisplaced distal medial or lateral malleolus fracture by immobilizing in weight-bearing short-leg cast or brace
   c. Nondisplaced bimalleolar fracture may require long-leg cast with knee flexed
   d. Displaced fractures may be reduced and held with closed management, but unstable or irreducible fractures best managed by ORIF to allow early motion
   e. After fracture heals, return to sports activity when 80–90% normal muscle strength regained

    f. In uncomplicated cases, return to practice within 3–6 mos, with
       return to preinjury status at 6–12 mos, depending on sport

Distal Tibial Physeal Fractures in the Adolescent

1. Mechanism of Injury: intra-articular fracture results from forces that
    cause supination-external rotation and pronation-external rotation
    fracture patterns in adults
2. Radiographic Evaluation
    a. Plain radiographs not adequate for proper evaluation (Fig. 22–7A)
    b. Accurate assessment of fracture configuration and displacement
      requires CT (Fig. 22–7B)

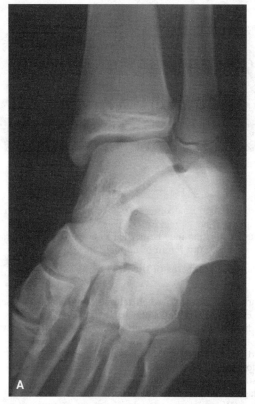

Fig. 22–7. A. A fairly benign-looking fracture of the epiphysis of the distal
tibia. B. CT of the same individual shows 4–5 mm displacement. This degree
of displacement is associated with significant risk of post-traumatic arthrosis.

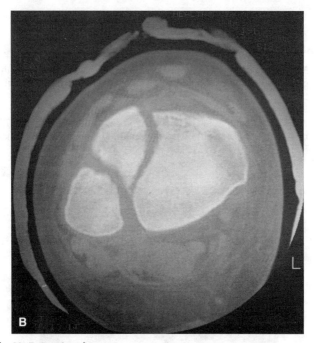

Fig. 22–7. *(continued).*

3. Treatment
   a. Reduce easily, but often difficult to hold to < 2 mm residual displacement
   b. Internal fixation may be needed to properly stabilize fracture
   c. Healing and full return of normal function in 3–6 mos

Osteochondral Fractures of the Ankle

1. Mechanism of Injury
   a. Part of ankle sprain when talus, tilting out of mortise, strikes lateral or medial malleolus
   b. Articular surface of joint affected, with fracture in most lateral or medial (more posterior) margin of talar dome
   c. Articular portion of fibula or medial malleolus can sustain osteochondral injury
2. Classification: based on radiographic appearance
   a. Stage I: compression fracture
   b. Stage II: partial osteochondral fragment separation
   c. Stage III: complete fragment separation and displacement
   d. Stage IV: displaced osteochondral fracture

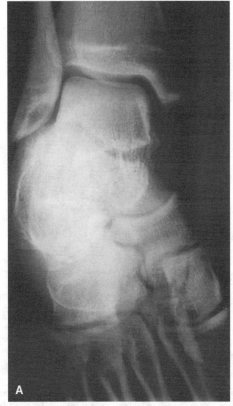

Fig. 22–8. A. A normal mortise view showed no abnormalities in the talus of this patient with chronic pain. B. The patient underwent MRI, which revealed a lateral talar osteochondral injury.

3. Clinical Presentation
   a. Unexplained chronic ankle pain after sprain
   b. Activity-related pain, swelling, joint catching, weakness, or joint instability for mos or yrs
4. Radiographic Evaluation
   a. Plain films often show no abnormality (Fig. 22–8A)
   b. Bone scan or MRI identifies fracture (Fig. 22–8B)
5. Treatment
   a. None for asymptomatic, nondisplaced lesions
   b. Immobilize symptomatic Stage I and II and medial Stage III fractures in short-leg cast for 6–8 wks

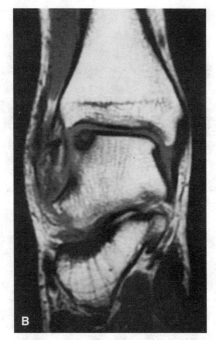

Fig. 22–8. *(continued).*

    c. Surgically excise Stage IV and lateral Stage III lesions
    d. Surgically excise other lesions symptomatic despite immobilization
    e. Perform surgery by open arthrotomy or arthroscopic technique

Fractures of the Posterior Process of the Talus

1. Mechanism of Injury
    a. Direct posterior process compression between calcaneus and tibia during forced plantar flexion (Fig. 22–9), which can occur acutely or from repeated trauma
    b. Can occur as avulsion of posterior talofibular ligament during inversion injury
    c. Most common site: posterior process lateral tubercle
2. Clinical Presentation
    a. Deep posterolateral ankle pain aggravated by forced plantar flexion activities of foot (eg, downhill walking or running)

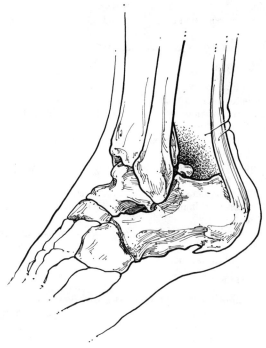

Fig. 22–9. A rendition of a posterior os trigonum-type fracture shows how, on forced plantar flexion, the posterior process can be squeezed between the posterior margin of the tibia and the posterior edge of the subtalar joint on the calcaneus.

    b. Tenderness over posterior talus
    c. Pain with resisted flexor hallucis longus function or forced plantar
       flexion
3. Radiographic Evaluation
    a. Lateral film best demonstrates fracture
    b. Acute fracture has irregular fracture margins
    c. Obtain bone scan if diagnosis still in question
4. Treatment
    a. Conservative: immobilize for 4–6 wks, and avoid weight bearing
       on acute fractures
    b. If symptoms persist, surgical excision warranted; after surgery,
       return to activity within 1–3 mos

Talar Neck Fractures

1. Mechanism of Injury: high-energy trauma

2. Treatment
   a. Anatomic reduction needed to avoid subtalar mechanism disruption
   b. Significant risk of avascular necrosis

Subtalar Dislocations

1. Mechanism of Injury
   a. Medial or lateral dislocation
   b. Medial dislocation: result of inversion injury (basketball foot)
2. Clinical Presentation: foot obviously dislocated, often with severe skin tenting across talar head
3. Treatment
   a. Prompt reduction under anesthesia to avert necrosis from skin tension
   b. Closed reduction sufficient for most cases
   c. Short period of immobilization (2–3 wks) to avoid subtalar joint stiffness
   d. Return to normal function at 6–8 wks if strength and comfort level adequate
   e. Strap foot for practice and competition for 6–9 mos

Plantar Fascia Rupture

1. Mechanism of Injury: seen in athletes with previous symptoms or treatment for plantar fasciitis (particularly if treated with multiple corticosteroid injections)
2. Clinical Presentation
   a. Sudden, severe heel pain following intense activity
   b. Localized tenderness and swelling
   c. As swelling ↓, palpable defect at site of lesion
   d. Ecchymosis in arch
3. Treatment
   a. Avoid weight bearing, use crutches, and ice for 15 mins 3 times/day until symptoms subside (usually in 2 wks)
   b. Once pain resolves, begin gradual weight bearing
   c. Provide support with pad or soft orthotic in shoe and with taping
   d. Crutches until full weight bearing and normal walking possible
   e. Full return to activity when able to stand on tiptoe without pain (usually within 3–6 wks)
   f. If conservative measures fail, surgical transection of plantar fascia may be necessary

Dislocation of the Peroneal Tendons

1. Mechanism of Injury: peroneal retinaculum may be injured by forceful peroneal tendon contraction on dorsiflexed foot
2. Clinical Presentation
   a. Acute injury

(1) Within few hrs, lateral ankle swelling indistinguishable from that of ankle sprain

(2) Once swelling severe, may be difficult to recognize tendency of tendons to move in and out of normal position

(3) Painful ankle motion, similar to ankle sprain

(4) Major differentiating feature: site of maximal tenderness
  (a) With ankle sprain, worst pain anterior to fibula
  (b) With peroneal tendon dislocation, maximal tenderness posteriorly

b. Chronic recurrent subluxation

(1) Recurrent ankle pain and/or instability

(2) Painful joint popping

(3) Observe and palpate tendon dislocation by having patient evert foot against resistance in plantar flexion and dorsiflexion

3. Radiographic Evaluation: normally shows no bony injury, though occasionally avulsion fracture of fibular posterior lip seen

4. Treatment: surgical repair for both acute injury and symptomatic chronic dislocations

"Ankle Sprain" in Skeletally Immature Athlete

1. Mechanism of Injury: inversion trauma to ankle can avulse fibular epiphysis at growth plate (Fig. 22–10), sparing lateral ligaments

2. Clinical Presentation

a. Physeal fractures commonly misdiagnosed as ankle sprains because spontaneous reduction occurs and radiographs reveal no bony abnormalities

b. Make correct diagnosis by localizing site of maximum tenderness and swelling over distal fibular physis

3. Treatment

a. Immobilize with short-leg walking cast for 4 wks to minimize risk of displacement

b. Displaced fractures require reduction, possibly ORIF

c. Return to athletic activity when full pain-free ROM and strength restored, usually 6–8 wks after injury

TRAUMATIC INJURIES TO THE MIDFOOT

Lisfranc's Fracture

1. Mechanism of Injury

a. Tarsometatarsal joint injury can result from blow to back of heel with toes firmly planted to ground and foot plantar flexed (eg, football), during slide (eg, baseball), or in fall from en pointe or demi pointe position (eg, dancing)

b. As dorsal ligaments rupture, foot collapses into plantar flexion at tarsometatarsal joint

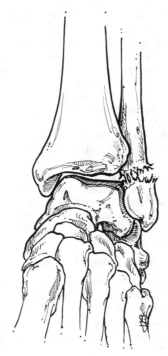

Fig. 22–10. An inversion injury to the ankle in an immature athlete can avulse the distal physis of the fibula.

       (1) Fractures of metatarsal and cuneiform bases frequent
       (2) Spontaneous reduction often occurs
2. Clinical Presentation
    a. Swelling may be severe or localized, even with significant injuries
    b. Tenderness along dorsal midfoot
    c. Pain with indirect stressing of joints
3. Radiographic Evaluation
    a. Lateral view: look for anatomic alignment of 1st metatarsal dorsal margin with lateral cuneiform
    b. AP view: look for perfect alignment of 2nd metatarsal medial edge and intermediate cuneiform
    c. Oblique view: look for same relationship for 3rd metatarsal and lateral cuneiform; also assess articulation of cuboid and 4th and 5th metatarsals
    d. Fractures of metatarsal bases, transverse base of 2nd metatarsal fractures, or cuboid fractures all suggest possible severe ligament injury

4. Treatment
   a. Anatomic reduction with internal fixation
   b. Recovery may take several mos

Jones Fracture

1. Mechanism of Injury: transverse fracture at proximal metaphyseal-diaphyseal junction of 5th metatarsal
2. Clinical and Radiographic Presentations
   a. Can present acutely: sudden onset of pain at time of injury, no prodromal symptoms, and radiographic signs consistent with acute injury
   b. With subacute fracture, mild discomfort precedes acute injury and radiographs show periosteal reaction
   c. Chronic form characterized by nonunion and intramedullary sclerosis
3. Treatment
   a. Immobilize acute fracture in weight-bearing or nonweight-bearing short-leg cast; union usually evident in 8–12 wks
   b. Treat subacute fractures same, but protracted healing may require surgery for union
   c. Chronic 5th metatarsal nonunion treated surgically by bone grafting or intramedullary screw fixation
   d. Significant risk of delayed union or nonunion, which can result in longterm disability, especially in athletes

Avulsion Fracture of the Tuberosity of the Fifth Metatarsal (Dancer's Fracture)

1. Mechanism of Injury: results when peroneus brevis muscle forcefully contracts during inversion injury, often avulsing insertion site at 5th metatarsal tuberosity (base)
2. Treatment
   a. Relieve symptoms and prevent severe fracture displacement
   b. Restrict athletic activity for at least 6 wks, with return to activity only after good (80%) eversion strength and full muscle control obtained
   c. Although nonunion common, fibrous healing usually asymptomatic and no treatment required

TRAUMATIC INJURIES TO THE FOREFOOT

Turf Toe

1. Mechanism of Injury: forced dorsiflexion of great toe metatarsophalangeal joint, jamming proximal phalanx against metatarsal head
2. Clinical Presentation
   a. Pain, tenderness, swelling, and painful joint motion
   b. Swelling and discomfort worsen during 24 hrs after injury

3. Radiographic Evaluation
    a. Capsular avulsion fracture of 1st metatarsal head or proximal phalanx base may be seen
    b. Sesamoid bone fractures can also be present
4. Treatment
    a. RICE and NSAIDs during acute phase
    b. No corticosteroid injections
    c. After acute phase: heat modalities, active and passive toe motion exercises, and foot-strengthening exercises
    d. Severe injuries take 3–6 wks to heal
    e. During rehab, tape toe or use stiff orthotic shoe insert to limit great toe dorsiflexion, relieve pain, and control swelling
    f. Return to activity when all symptoms resolve

Injury to the Great Toe Sesamoids

1. Mechanism of Injury
    a. Result of single acute episode, but more often no specific cause recalled
    b. Pain can be due to fracture, osteochondritis dissecans, sesamoiditis, bursitis, or callus beneath sesamoid
2. Clinical Presentation
    a. Pain in ball of foot with weight bearing, but exact location may be vague
    b. Significant sesamoid tenderness
3. Radiographic Evaluation
    a. Differentiating between undisplaced fracture and bipartite sesamoid difficult
    b. May see "mottled" appearance, cystic changes, or sesamoid collapse from osteochondritis dissecans (avascular necrosis)
4. Treatment
    a. Treat with rest and padding of area to relieve pressure
    b. If symptoms persist, sesamoid excision warranted
    c. Gradual return to activity approximately 6 wks after surgery

23

Overuse Injuries of the Lower Leg, Ankle, and Foot

MUSCLE STRAINS

Mechanism of Injury

1. Partial muscle-tendon unit disruptions result from forceful eccentric contractions
2. Disruption at musculotendinous junction followed by intense inflammatory reaction and subsequent fibrosis

Classification

1. 1st Degree: tear of few muscle or tendon fibers
2. 2nd Degree: disruption of moderate number of muscle or tendon fibers, but muscle-tendon unit remains intact
3. 3rd Degree: complete rupture of muscle-tendon unit

Clinical Presentation

1. 1st Degree Strain: strong, but painful muscle contraction
2. 2nd Degree Strain: moderate pain, swelling, and disability; able to produce only weak and painful attempt at muscle contraction
3. 3rd Degree Strain: extremely weak ability to produce muscle contraction

Treatment

1. Ice and elevation
2. Initiate gradual ROM exercises shortly after icing injured extremity
3. NSAIDs to relieve pain
4. Physical therapy modalities (eg, ultrasound, anaphoresis, electrical muscle stimulation)
5. Return to activity after pain and swelling subside and muscle strength and function sufficient for planned activity

SHIN SPLINTS

Mechanism of Injury

1. Cause of pain unknown, but may result from inflamed periosteum or avulsion of posteromedial distal tibial periosteum
2. Often noted in running athletes who change running surface, running technique, or shoe type

Clinical Presentation

Pain and tenderness localized to 6–10 cm immediately posterior to tibial ridge (Fig. 23–1)

Radiographic Evaluation

1. To rule out stress fracture
2. In chronic cases, posterior distal tibia may be mildly thickened or undulated
3. Bone scan usually normal or shows mild, diffuse uptake along painful area

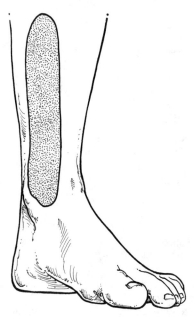

Fig. 23–1. Area of involvement in shin splints.

Treatment

1. Rest, duration depending on pain
2. NSAIDs of questionable benefit
3. Stretching and careful warm-up before athletic activity
4. Correct anatomic variations with semi-rigid foot orthosis
5. Use running shoe providing shock absorption and firm heel contour

ACHILLES TENDINITIS

Mechanism of Injury

Chronic, degenerative changes lead to inflammation, partial rupture, and tendinosis

Noninsertional Tendinitis

1. Clinical Presentation
   a. Pain 2–6 cm above Achilles tendon insertion, usually after exercise and often early in morning; as condition worsens, symptoms may occur during exercise or become constant
   b. Local thickening and tenderness along tendon
   c. Crepitus during acute phase of injury
   d. Reduced gastrocnemius-soleus flexibility: diminished ankle dorsiflexion with knee extended
   e. Paratenonitis may precede tendinosis (typically associated with chronic paratenonitis)
2. Radiographic Evaluation
   a. Routine radiographs not diagnostic, but may reveal tendon calcifications compatible with chronic degenerative changes
   b. Ultrasound: qualitative changes or partial tendon tears
   c. MRI: most accurate means of evaluating tendon, but reserved for tendinitis resistant to conservative treatment and for preoperative planning
3. Treatment
   a. Isolated Paratenonitis
      (1) Cease aggravating activity, rest, stretch, cold therapy, and orthotics to elevate heel or control pronation
      (2) NSAIDs provide pain relief during acute phase
      (3) No corticosteroid injections into tendon
      (4) For unresponsive cases, limited surgical approach to decompress tendon and lyse adhesions in paratenon worthwhile
   b. Tendinosis
      (1) Prognosis for recovery with conservative care less promising
      (2) If 4–6 mos conservative treatment fails to relieve pain, surgical intervention recommended
      (3) In severe cases, recovery slow, often ≥ 6–8 mos to return to intensive activity

Insertional Tendinitis

1. Clinical Presentation
   a. Symptoms localized to distal tendon, most often posterolaterally (tissue thickening evident); proximal tendon remains relatively normal
   b. Pain during or after exercise
   c. Focal erythema, warmth, and tenderness at insertion
   d. Gastrocnemius-soleus tightness
2. Radiographic Evaluation
   a. Spurs at insertion site on calcaneus, and occasionally calcification in distal tendon
   b. Abnormally prominent Haglund's process (Fig. 23–2)
   c. MRI may determine if 1° disorder is in tendon or adjacent tissues
3. Treatment
   a. Aimed at reducing tensile forces and contact pressures on distal Achilles tendon
   b. NSAIDs, cold therapy, and ultrasound
   c. Limited activity, with stretching and controlled strengthening exercises

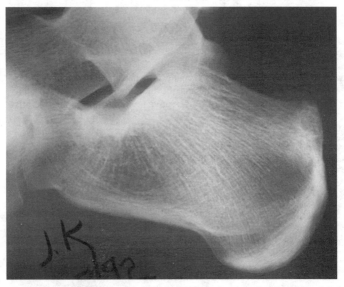

Fig. 23–2. Radiograph demonstrates chronic insertional tendinitis and reactive bone over Haglund's process.

    d. Cushion shoe's heel contour and add temporary heel lift
    e. When appropriate, orthotics limit pronation or accommodate other foot malalignments
    f. If retrocalcaneal or precalcaneal bursa contribute to chronic pain, careful corticosteroid injection into bursa tissue justified; avoid injection into tendon fibers
    g. If conservative treatment fails, consider surgical debridement of distal tendon and removal of prominent calcaneal process

ACHILLES TENDON RUPTURE

Mechanism of Injury

Strenuous activity results in forceful eccentric or concentric gastrocnemius-soleus contraction

Clinical Presentation

1. Abrupt, severe pain (as if kicked or struck) with no prodromal symptoms
2. Temporary severe pain
3. Prolonged limp with plantar flexion weakness if medical care postponed
4. Shortened stride from weakened push-off and inability to perform single-limb toe rise

Physical Examination

1. Thompson's Test (Fig. 23–3)
    a. Most reliable test for tendon rupture
    b. Patient lies prone with feet suspended in air
    c. Firmly squeeze calf; if no passive movement of ankle and foot cannot be plantar flexed, complete rupture probable
2. Palpable defect in tendon also confirms rupture

Radiographic Evaluation

1. Radiographs not helpful in diagnosis, but useful for evaluating associated disorders (eg, rare avulsion fracture off posterior calcaneal tuberosity)
2. MRI and ultrasound assess tendon apposition when choosing nonsurgical treatment or evaluating late or chronic ruptures

Treatment

1. Nonsurgical Treatment
    a. Generally successful, but higher risk of re-rupture within 6 mos of injury
    b. Prolonged immobilization in equinus ↑ rehab time
    c. Most successful when initiated within 48 hrs of injury
    d. Place foot in "forced plantar flexion" in short-leg cast for 4 wks, followed by 4 wks of "semiequinus" casting

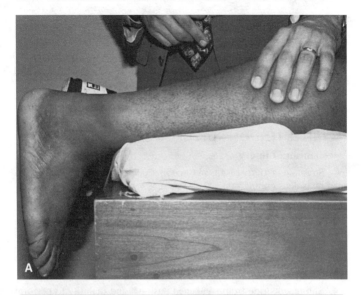

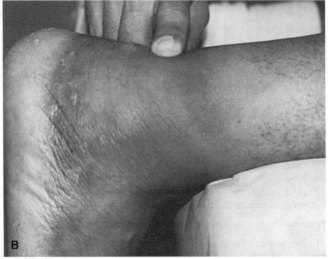

Fig. 23–3. A. A positive Thompson's test associated with a ruptured Achilles tendon: the foot cannot be plantar flexed with this maneuver. B. Identification of a palpable defect in the typical location of Achilles rupture.

    e. Use heel raise for 4 wks after cast removal, followed by progressive rehab exercises
2. Surgical Treatment
    a. Surgical apposition of ruptured tendon ends: most consistent means of regaining gastrocnemius-soleus power
    b. Some techniques allow casting in neutral position or permit limited early ankle ROM
    c. Surgically treated patients achieve earlier return to functional activity and avoid prolonged process of regaining ankle dorsiflexion associated with equinus casting
    d. Re-rupture risk considerably lower in surgically repaired tendons
3. Postoperative Management
    a. When early ROM possible, use dorsiflexion block splint or removable protective brace
    b. Often cast protection for 4–6 wks is best
    c. Touch-down weight bearing necessary during first 3–4 wks
    d. Then, gradually ↑ to full weight bearing in cast or protective brace
    e. All surgical repairs require cast or brace protection for at least 6–8 wks
    f. Start progressive resistive exercises and continue regaining ankle flexibility
    g. Most patients return to sports activity 4–6 mos after surgery

HEEL PAIN

Heel Bruise

1. Mechanism of Injury: often seen in foot with very mobile fat pad
2. Physical Examination: medial calcaneal tubercle tenderness
3. Treatment
    a. Pulsed ultrasound ↓ inflammation and point stimulation ↓ pain
    b. Manual fat pad massage lyses adhesions
    c. Heel cup absorbs shock
    d. Corticosteroid injection if conservative treatment fails; however, fat necrosis can occur

Heel Pad Trauma

1. Mechanism of Injury: repetitive heel pad trauma flattens and spreads fat and septa, decreasing shock-absorbing ability
2. Clinical Presentation: morning pain improves shortly after activity begins

Calcaneal Stress Fractures

1. Mechanism of Injury: Inactive persons who suddenly start vigorous sports activity or athletes who suddenly ↑ training intensity or duration
2. Clinical Presentation
   a. Sharp, persistent, progressive pain or deep, dull ache over calcaneus
   b. Impact pain
   c. Elicit pain by squeezing medial and lateral calcaneal borders
   d. Point tenderness, plantar calcaneus
3. Radiographic Evaluation
   a. Lateral view and special lateral view at 45° best
   b. Bone scan more specific for early fracture detection
4. Treatment
   a. Rest and cease sports activity until fracture heals
   b. May use short-leg cast immobilization for protection and comfort
   c. Weight bear and return to activity only when pain resolves

PLANTAR FASCIITIS

Mechanism of Injury

Periosteal avulsion, microtear, or fascial inflammation at insertion at medial calcaneal tubercle on os calcis plantar surface (Fig. 23–4)

Clinical Presentation

1. Sharp heel pain, usually at medial process of calcaneal tuberosity
2. Pain may lessen with activity or be felt as burning sensation or dull ache during activity
3. Weight bearing exacerbates pain
4. Swelling rare
5. Most cases unilateral

Physical Examination

1. Fascial tautness
2. Limited dorsiflexion indicates ↓ flexibility (ie, tight Achilles tendon)
3. Elicit pain by passively stretching fascia and Achilles tendon, dorsiflexing foot, or having patient stand on toes

Radiographic Evaluation

1. Spur formation in 50% of cases, but not cause of pain
2. Bone scan or MRI can help

Treatment

1. Rest and NSAIDs
2. Heel cord stretching exercises

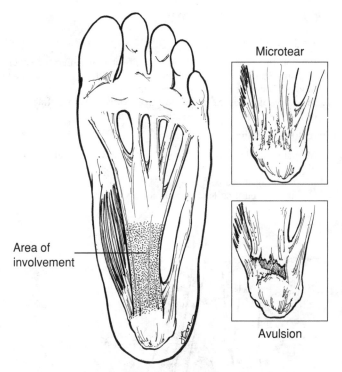

Fig. 23–4. Disorders at the insertion of the plantar fascia at the calcaneal medial tubercle on the plantar surface of the os calcis that can cause plantar fasciitis include periosteal avulsion, microtear, and inflammation of the fascia.

3. Train on soft surfaces (eg, grass)
4. Ice for 20–30 mins after athletic activity
5. Soft orthotic with Tuli heel cup
6. Consider corrective orthotics for varus or pronation biomechanical foot anomaly
7. Ankle-foot orthotic night splints with 5° dorsiflexion for refractory cases
8. Slow and gradual improvement over 1 yr
9. Corticosteroid injection into medial tubercle may be justified if conservative treatment unsuccessful, but repeated injections can rupture plantar fascia or atrophy heel pad
10. As last resort, consider surgical release of plantar fascia, but results vary significantly

TARSAL TUNNEL SYNDROME

Mechanism of Injury

1. Entrapment: posterior tibial nerve in flexor retinaculum or either or both branches (ie, medial and lateral plantar nerves) as they traverse abductor hallucis muscle (Fig. 23–5)
2. Most common causes in athletes: heel varus or valgus, fractures, dislocations, and direct pressure (os trigonum)

Clinical Presentation

1. Medial malleolus pain radiating to sole of foot, heel, and occasionally up calf and leg
   a. Poorly localized pain
   b. Runners: burning heel pain or aching in arch

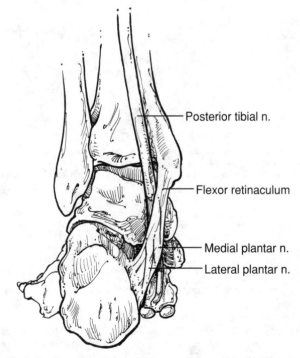

Fig. 23–5. Tarsal tunnel syndrome due to entrapment within the flexor retinaculum of the posterior tibial nerve, or either or both of its branches (ie, medial and lateral plantar nerves).

    c. Activity exacerbates pain and causes longitudinal arch cramping
    d. Night pain
    e. Removing shoes or elevating feet relieves pain
2. Paresthesia, dysesthesia, and hyperesthesia
3. Burning or numbness of plantar foot or toes
4. Sensory loss in medial or plantar nerve distribution
5. Swelling over course of posterior tibial nerve from space-occupying lesion

Physical Examination

1. Note excessive varus or valgus heel, excessive external rotation of foot, or high arch
2. Tinel's sign over posterior tibial nerve or abductor hallucis
3. Dorsiflexion, inversion, or eversion may reproduce symptoms
4. Tenderness over abductor hallucis or proximal or distal to posterior tibial nerve
5. Pain relief following corticosteroid-Xylocaine injection directly into tarsal tunnel confirms diagnosis

Radiographic Evaluation

1. AP, lateral, and oblique views delineate soft tissue masses, bony anomalies, or traumatic disorders creating space-occupying lesion
2. Perform MRI if mass suspected

Treatment

1. Rest, ice, NSAIDs, change shoe wear, correct shoe tightness, additional arch support, and orthotics to correct abnormal foot mechanics
2. Consider corticosteroid-Xylocaine injection
3. If conservative measures unsuccessful, may need surgical decompression of tarsal tunnel

STRESS FRACTURES OF THE FOREFOOT

Metatarsal Stress Fracture

1. Mechanism of Injury: repetitive loading causes bone failure and shaft fracture
2. Clinical Presentation
    a. Pain, with limping on weight bearing
    b. Swelling
3. Radiographic Evaluation: fracture may not be evident until wks after injury, when new bone forms
4. Treatment
    a. Rest and limited weight bearing
    b. Crutches often sufficient, but may need cast immobilization if pain significant

    c. Pain may persist 2–3 wks and healing may require 6–8 wks
    d. Return to activity when all symptoms abate and radiographs show good healing
    e. Rigid protective footwear during initial return to sports activity

Sesamoid Stress Fracture

1. Mechanism of Injury: excessive functional overload
2. Clinical Presentation: localized sesamoid pain exacerbated by weight bearing or palpation
3. Radiographic Evaluation: visible fracture may persist as fibrous union
4. Treatment
    a. Rest and splint
    b. Donut orthotic to protect pressure point
    c. Cast rarely necessary
    d. Return to sports activity gradually
    e. Shoe insert to splint great toe
    f. Chronic cases may need surgery to debride or repair nonhealing sesamoid fracture

REACTIVE SYNOVITIS OF THE FOREFOOT

Metatarsalgia

1. Mechanism of Injury: ↑ weight-bearing pressure irritates soft tissue about metatarsal head and causes callus buildup
2. Treatment
    a. Relieve inflammation with foot soaks and NSAIDs
    b. Examine footwear for focal pressure points; redistribute focal pressure with special shoe insert to lift prominent metatarsal head or orthotic insert cut out to accommodate callus
    c. Trim calluses
    d. Orthotics provide cushioning beneath metatarsal heads to prevent recurrence

Neuritis

1. Mechanism of Injury
    a. Irritation and resultant inflammation of intermetatarsal nerves as they become digital sensory nerves
    b. Progresses to fibrosis, and then vasculitis, which can stimulate scar tissue formation about nerve
2. Treatment
    a. In early stages: rest, soaks, protective padding, and NSAIDs
    b. Corticosteroid injections may resolve inflammation
    c. Chronic neuromas, however, respond poorly to conservative therapy, cause significant pain and functional disability, and should be surgically removed

Bracing and Taping for Prevention and Treatment of Injuries

PROPHYLACTIC KNEE BRACES

Design Concept

1. Protect knee from injury or reduce injury severity by absorbing direct or indirect stress placed on knee during athletic maneuver
2. Ideal prophylactic knee brace would ↓ severity and frequency of disabling knee injuries without affecting normal speed and agility

Types of Prophylactic Knee Braces

1. Lateral bar-based hinged designs fitted with hyperextension stop (Fig. 24–1)
   a. Early protective braces (lateral-based, hinged supports) developed to minimize force of direct contact lateral blows to knees and redirect force above and below
   b. These braces intended to statically restrain abnormal knee motion, especially in response to valgus stress
   c. Designed to protect medial collateral ligament (MCL) from direct contact valgus blow
2. Medial and lateral-based designs incorporate plastic cuff or strap-suspension system with medial and lateral supports held together with polycentric hinge
   a. Theoretically, newer designs ↓ absolute strain on knee ligaments by dissipating impact forces above and below joint and by ↑ duration of impact loading
   b. Manufacturers contend that they protect other ligaments, including ACL, in both contact and noncontact injuries
   c. Many braces used also as functional or rehabilitative braces

Current Indications

1. Inconclusive evidence that prophylactic knee bracing ↓ rate or severity of knee injuries, and in fact, may ↑ risk of injury

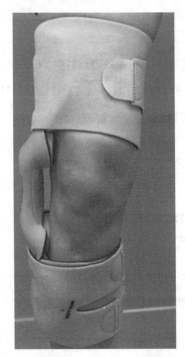

Fig. 24–1. The Anderson Knee stabler (Omni Scientific, Concord, CA).

2. Thus, AAOS and American Academy of Pediatrics do not recommend prophylactic knee braces at this time

REHABILITATIVE KNEE BRACES

Design Concept

1. Developed from principle of splinting or casting injured ligaments to allow adequate healing; based on studies showing improved ligamentous healing of knee injuries when motion over controlled arc maintained
2. Allows protected motion of injured knee during healing, whether treated surgically or nonsurgically, while preventing abnormal varus or valgus stress
3. Design includes medial and lateral support arms, hinge system to allow knee motion, thigh and calf enclosures incorporating straps for

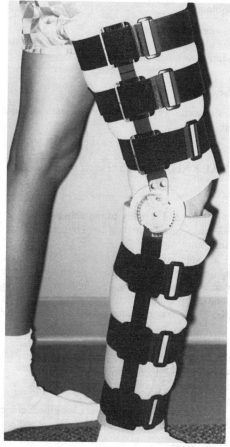

Fig. 24–2. Vantage long-leg brace (Vantage Orthopaedics, Cincinnati, OH).

support and suspension, and often flexion and extension stops to limit arc of motion (Fig. 24–2)

Advantages

1. Easy application and removal, comfort, lightweight protection, static stability, and off-the-shelf accessibility
2. Ease in obtaining postoperative knee motion, lower rates of ankylosis, and less frequent need for subsequent knee manipulation

Potential Problems

1. Dependent edema below brace straps
2. Fitting difficulties for severe angular deformities or leg size extremes
3. Improper fitting or hinge placement
4. Limited means of ensuring compliance with brace wear

Current Indications

Rehab braces well accepted by injured athletes, facilitate early aggressive rehab

FUNCTIONAL KNEE BRACES

Design Concept

1. Provide protection and stability to unstable knee and allow athlete to continue participating at highest level by minimizing pain, swelling, and instability
2. Minimize absolute displacement or rotation of tibia on femur by preventing hyperextension and ↑ resistance to displacement
3. Other possible mechanisms: augment limb proprioception and alter limb position during cutting maneuvers, which ideally should prevent or minimize giving way episodes associated with pivot shift

Types of Functional Braces

1. Hinge-post-strap design: Prototype was brace originally designed to control anteromedial rotatory instability in Joe Namath's knee (Fig. 24–3)
2. Hinge-post-shell design (Fig. 24–4A–C)
   a. Semi-rigid plastic shell encompasses both thigh and calf
   b. Developed to improve soft-tissue contact area and brace suspension
   c. Other possible benefits: ↑ brace stiffness and rigidity

Brace Effectiveness

1. In vitro studies: effective at controlling anteroposterior translation at very low loads, but may be limited in controlling knee laxity when joint subjected to forceful stresses of athletic activities
2. Brace does not return athlete to "normal," so not adequate substitute for reconstructive surgery in competitive athlete who wants to maintain highest level of function
3. However, athletes report high level of satisfaction, subjectively noting ↓ instability symptoms, pain relief, and sense of protection from brace wear

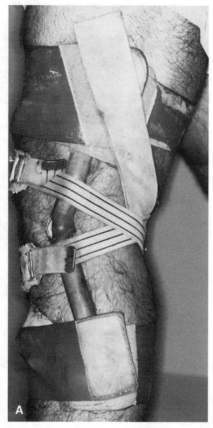

Fig. 24–3. The Lenox Hill derotation brace (Lenox Hill Brace Shop, New York, NY).

4. Functional bracing may also be effective after ACL reconstruction by reducing repetitive loads on ACL graft

Current Indications

1. Use postoperatively, as surgery substitute, and prophylactically
2. Use in nonsurgically treated patients with unstable knees to ↓ frequency of instability episodes
3. Use in patients with knee instability secondary to neuromuscular disease that precludes surgical stabilization

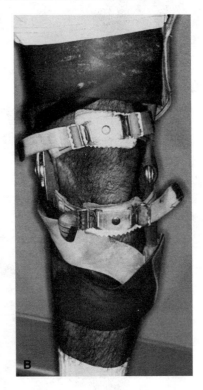

Fig. 24–3. *(continued).*

4. Brace use after knee ligament reconstruction remains controversial, ranging from
   a. Wearing brace during all subsequent sporting activities
   b. Wearing only during 1st yr after surgery to allow grafted ligament to mature
   c. Using only when surgery produces suboptimal results and residual instability remains

Limitations

1. No clear evidence that braces protect injured or reconstructed knees from further injury or minimize post-traumatic arthritis
2. Current braces adversely affect speed and agility and ↑ energy consumption, which may make knee more vulnerable to further injury
3. Athletes frequently complain of brace migration and slipping during sporting activities
4. Other problems: improper fitting and loss of suspension

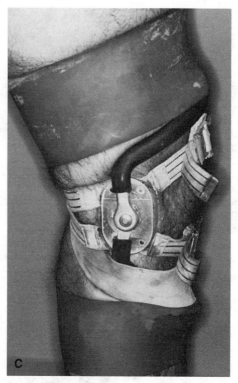

Fig. 24–3. *(continued).*

PATELLOFEMORAL BRACES

Design Concept

1. Primary goal: diminish symptomatic lateral patellar subluxation by mechanically ↓ lateral patellar displacement
2. Other potential benefits: warming effect on knee and reduced swelling
3. Most constructed of neoprene or elastic sleeve, frequently combined with buttress pad or strapping system for additional support (Fig. 24–5)

Current Indications

Adjunct only to rehab program that includes strengthening and flexibility exercises

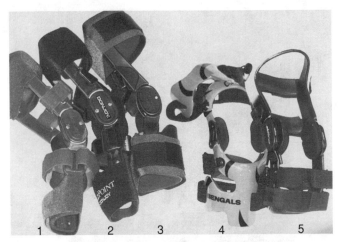

Fig. 24–4. Common functional knee braces: (1) 4-Point brace (DonJoy, Carlsbad, CA); (2) Gold Point (DonJoy); (3) Bledsoe Force Brace (Medical Technology, Grand Prairie, TX); (4) CTI 2 (Innovation Sports, Irvine, CA); (5) Defiance (DonJoy).

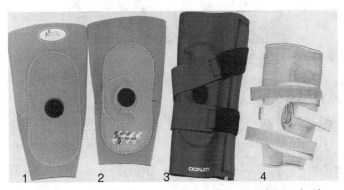

Fig. 24–5. Common patellar braces: (1, 2) Sports supports without and with lateral support (The Sports Medicine Co., Irvine, TX); (3) lateral patellar knee support (DonJoy); (4) Palumbo patellar stabilizing brace (Dynorthotics, Vienna, VA).

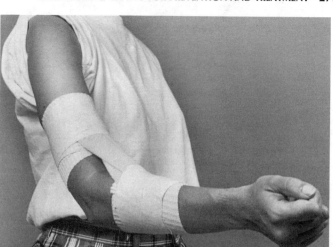

Fig. 24–6. Hyperextension of the elbow can be prevented by placing anchor straps on the upper arm and forearm, and using several strips placed over the front of the elbow with the joint flexed to act as a checkrein.

TAPING AND WRAPPING

General Guidelines

1. Shave areas to be taped to prevent hair loss and skin irritation
2. Tape adherent ensures that tape sticks and protects skin
3. Underwrap decreases friction where skin very tender, but may reduce stabilizing effect of taping
4. If prewrap insufficient, use grease pads or another lubricant to prevent blisters

Shoulder

1. Clavicle fractures: Use elastic bandage to form **X**, pulling shoulders back
2. Acromioclavicular (AC) joint sprains: Place overlapping strips along clavicle and AC joint to stabilize joint (place pad over nipple to prevent irritating friction)

Elbow

1. To protect from hyperextension, place anchor strips above and below joint
2. Bend elbow short of position where pain begins
3. Place 2–3 strips of tape (directly on top of each other or in **X**) on

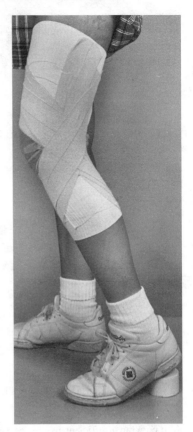

Fig. 24–7. Taping to stabilize the knee after a medial or lateral sprain should include several strips forming an X over the sides of the knee, to protect it from varus and valgus forces.

top of anchor strips at both ends, with additional anchor strips over overlapping strips (Fig. 24–6)

Wrist, Hand, and Fingers

1. Support wrist by taping either around wrist or in X over dorsal or plantar surface of hand
2. Support finger by buddy taping (taping adjacent fingers together)
3. Stabilize thumb with figure-of-eight pattern, adding strips to prevent abduction and adduction

Hip and Thigh

1. Hamstrings and quadriceps strains: Wrap 6-inch-wide elastic bandage around upper leg to control swelling and provide support

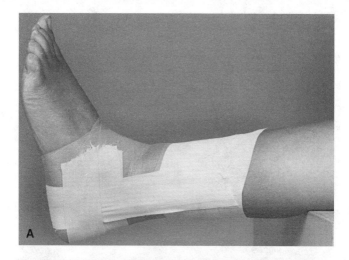

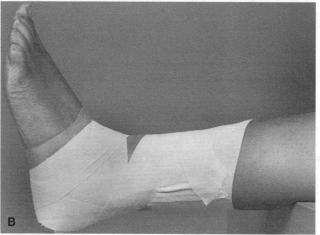

Fig. 24–8. A. Basic taping to support the ankle includes anchor strips at the musculotendinous junction of the Achilles tendon and gastrocnemius, followed by three stirrups and three Gibney straps. B. After heel locks are added, a figure-of-eight should be applied, to prevent excessive plantar flexion. C. Finally, strips of tape should be placed to cover the stirrups and to help stabilize the ankle joint.

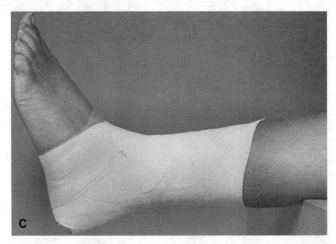

Fig. 24–8. *(continued).*

2. Groin pull
   a. With 6-inch-wide elastic wrap, start at distal thigh and rotate upward, going from medial to lateral
   b. Continue to wrap hip to ensure proper support and prevent wrap from slipping down thigh

Knee

1. Medial and lateral sprains

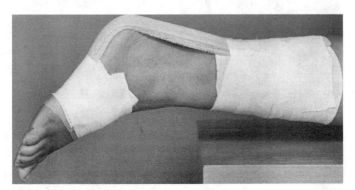

Fig. 24–9. Taping for a patient with an Achilles tendon injury should keep the foot positioned in plantar flexion, to prevent premature stretching of the tendon.

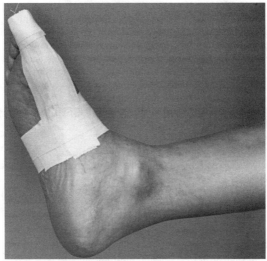

Fig. 24–10. For the athlete with turf toe, the taping should stabilize the great toe to prevent hyperextension.

    a. Place several anchor strips above and below joint; then, alternate strips of tape in X fashion over medial or lateral side to protect from varus and valgus forces (Fig. 24–7)
    b. Apply rotation strip, if necessary, and finally, anchor strips over other strips to ensure attachment
2. Hyperextension
    a. Place anchor strips above and below joint
    b. Place patch in popliteal area to prevent friction and irritation
    c. Then alternate strips to form X over posterior knee, followed by anchor strips (again) above and below joint to strengthen attachment

Lower Leg, Ankle, and Foot

1. Shin splints: Starting distally, overlap strips of tape, going from lateral to medial around calf (elastic tape best: allows muscles to expand)
2. Ankle sprains
    a. Overlap 3 anchor strips at Achilles tendon-gastrocnemius junction, followed by 3 stirrups and 3 Gibney straps alternated posterior and inferior to lateral malleolus (Fig. 24–8)
    b. Heel locks (one on each side) ensure stability
    c. Figure-of-eight prevents excessive plantar flexion
    d. Cover stirrups with strips of tape

3. Achilles tendon injuries
   a. Place one anchor strip at Achilles tendon-gastrocnemius junction, along with anchor strips at midfoot
   b. Plantar flex foot to prevent premature tendon stretching
   c. Place 2–3 strips of elastic tape at base of foot, and with slight pulling action, attach other ends to calf anchor strip (Fig. 24–9)
   d. Split tape from heel to top of musculotendinous junction, providing end pieces to wrap around anterior shin
   e. Place several anchor strips over calf and foot to ensure proper attachment
4. Longitudinal Arch
   a. Place anchor strip around distal foot
   b. Alternate strips of tape (usually 6–8) from medial to lateral with foot relaxed
   c. Finally, place several strips from lateral to medial along plantar foot
5. Turf toe
   a. Place anchor strips around forefoot and great toe
   b. Starting from great toe, place strips of tape to forefoot anchor strip, each strip overlapping, until toe stabilized
   c. Finally, place additional anchor strips around great toe and forefoot (Fig. 24–10)

Rehabilitation of Athletic Injuries

PRIMARY FOCUS

Functional outcome (rapid return of athlete to competition) rather than simply treatment of symptoms

THERAPEUTIC MODALITIES

Most effective when combined with exercise in rehab program

CRYOTHERAPY (THERAPEUTIC COOLING)

1. General Concepts
   a. Occurs through conduction or evaporation
   b. Ice massage produces more cooling than gel pack
   c. Greater the temperature difference between skin and cooling source, greater the resulting change in temperature
   d. Longer the treatment, greater the resulting change in temperature
2. Indications: acute and chronic sprains, strains, contusions, fractures, minor burns and abrasions, heat illness, acute phase of inflammatory bursitis, tendinitis, tenosynovitis, and muscle spasms
3. Forms of Treatment
   a. Apply ice packs or gel packs directly to skin for 15–30 min, checking skin every 20 min to prevent frostbite
   b. Terry cloth chilled in bucket of crushed ice and water useful, but must be changed every 4–5 min
   c. Ice massage
      (1) To ice small, superficial area of inflammation (eg, elbow epicondyles, patellar tendon, knee collateral ligaments, and ankle ligaments), massage with ice cube in circular motion for 5–10 min until area numb
      (2) Also use ice massage over muscle for up to 15 min, both

285

for contusion and for reducing muscle spasms (eg, back and hamstrings)

d. Immerse larger areas in bucket of cold water and ice (temperature range 12.5–26°C)
   (1) 10–20 min to control swelling
   (2) For pain relief, until anesthesia produced

4. Vapocoolant Sprays (fluoromethane, ether chloride)
   a. Rapidly cool area for analgesic effect
   b. Convenient for acute muscle spasms
      (1) Stretch muscle as far as comfortable and spray unidirectionally
      (2) Hold spray 2 ft from muscle and move 4 in/sec, covering muscle at least twice
      (3) After spraying, apply additional force and gently stretch muscle
      (4) Warm skin with hands and repeat treatment up to 3 times

5. Precautions
   a. Do not apply cold too soon after injury (may ↑ swelling)
   b. Do not use too cold temperatures
   c. Do not apply cold for > 30 min
   d. Do not apply cold directly over superficial nerve

6. Contraindications: Cardiac dysfunction (including angina pectoris); open wounds older than 48–72 hrs; arterial insufficiency; cold hypersensitivity; peripheral neuropathies, including diabetes

Compression

1. Combine Ace bandage or Tubigrip (Fig. 25–1) with ice pack for compression
2. Keep compressive wrap on at all times during first several days to control swelling, then use only during day
3. Combine compression and cryotherapy in devices such as Cryocuff (Fig. 25-2) or Cryotemp

Ultrasound (US)

1. Pulsed US
   a. Use low-intensity pulsed US during early inflammation when heating contraindicated
   b. Divide area into treatment zones measuring $1\frac{1}{2}$ times effective radiating area (ERA)
   c. For acute injury, treat each zone 1–2 min
   d. Frequency: 3MHz for superficial tissue, 1MHz for deeper tissue
   e. Move sound head slowly over affected area in overlapping circular motion

2. Continuous US
   a. Indicated when selective tissue (eg, tendon, cartilage, ligament,

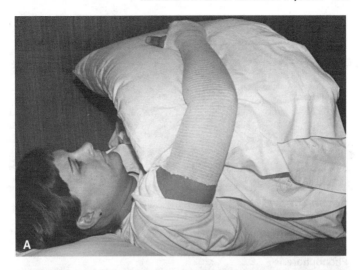

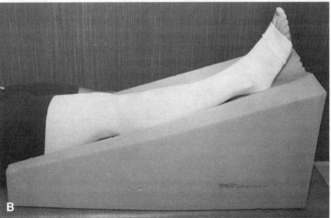

Fig. 25–1. Tubigrip is easy for the patient to use at home and comes in various sizes to fit (A) the arm or (B) the leg.

bone) heating desired to facilitate stretching of contracted deep connective tissue
  b. Does not heat highly vascularized tissue (eg, muscle)
    (1) Rather, circulation ↑ to dissipate heat
    (2) Local blood flow ↑ significantly, which may help in tissue healing and treating muscle spasms

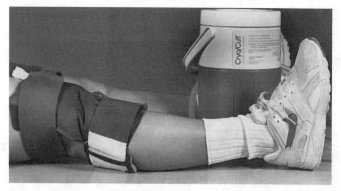

Fig. 25–2. The Cryocuff uses a thermos of ice and water, which can be raised to different heights to control the amount of pressure in the cuff.

Phonophoresis

1. Topical application of anti-inflammatory medications with US to control inflammation
2. Most commonly used medications: hydrocortisone cream (0.5%, 1%, 5%, or 10% concentration) and salicylate (Myoflex cream)

Iontophoresis

1. Electric current introduces soluble salt ions into body tissues for therapeutic purposes
2. Dexamethasone sodium phosphate (most common medication) used for acute inflammation, but more often for chronic inflammation (other useful medications in Table 25–1)
3. Better release of medications and improved safety from advances in buffering medications and in electrode material and adding buffering agent to electrode (Fig. 25–3)
4. Treatment protocol
   a. May be used for single visit or 4–6 treatments with exercises and bracing
   b. Current based on patient's tolerance to sensation when activated (base setting: 2.0 mA)
   c. Treat 15–20 min depending on medication dose
   d. Wipe clean with alcohol skin area where medicated and ground pads placed
   e. Saturate medicated pad with 1mL dexamethasone (depending on machine used)
   f. Patient feels mild tingling sensation once treatment starts; if sensation too intense, reduce current

Table 25–1. Currently Used Ions: Properties and Sources

Hydrocortisone: 1% ointment, various local sources, positive pole; anti-inflammatory; avoid ointments with ''paraben'' preservatives; used for arthritis, tendinitis, myositis, bursitis

Mecholyl: mecholyl ointment, (Gordon Labs, Upper Darby, PA); positive pole; vasodilator, analgesic; used for neuritis, neurovascular deficits, sprains, edema

Lidocaine: from Xylocaine 5% (Astra Pharmaceutical Co., Westboro, MA); positive pole; anesthetic analgesic; used for neuritis, bursitis, painful range of motion

Acetic acid: 10% stock solution, cut to 2%; negative pole; used for calcific deposits, myositis ossificans, frozen joints

Iodine: from Iodex (with methyl salicylate); negative pole; sclerolytic, antiseptic, analgesic; used for scar tissue, adhesions, fibrositis

Salicylate: from Myoflex (Adria Labs, Columbus, OH) ointment, 10% salicylate preparation, or Iodex *with* methyl salicylate (Medtech Labs Inc., Cody, WY); negative pole; decongestant, analgesic; used for myalgias, rheumatoid arthritis

Magnesium: from 2% solution of magnesium sulfate (Epsom salts); positive pole; antispasmodic, analgesic, vasodilator; used for osteoarthritis, myositis, neuritis

Copper: 2% solution, copper sulfate; positive pole; caustic, antiseptic, antifungal; used for allergic rhinitis, dermatophytosis (athlete's foot)

Zinc: from zinc oxide ointment 20%; positive pole; caustic, antiseptic; enhances healing; used for otitis, ulcerations, dermatitis, other open lesions

Calcium: from calcium chloride, 2% solution; positive pole; stabilizer or irritability threshold; used for myospasm, frozen joints, trigger finger, mild tremors (non-Parkinsonian)

Chlorine: from table salt (NaCl), 2% solution; negative pole; sclerolytic; used for scar tissue, adhesions

Lithium: from lithium chloride or lithium carbonate, 2% solution; positive pole; specifically for gouty tophi

Hyaluronidase: from Wydase (Wyeth, Philadelphia, PA); solution to be mixed as directed on vials; positive pole; absorption agent for edema, sprains

(Kahn, J.: Principles and Practice of Electrotherapy. 3rd Ed. New York, Churchill Livingstone, 1994. p. 138.)

Electrical Stimulation

1. Apply high-voltage pulsed current (HVPC) at 120 pulses per sec (pps) and 90% intensity to produce muscle contraction to injured area for up to 4 30-min treatments within 8 hrs of injury

2. Beneficial where muscle function inhibited after knee injury (particularly patellar dislocation), or in postop knees

3. Suggested treatment protocol in absence of active muscle contraction
   a. Use muscle-stimulating device with frequency around 2500 Hz adjustable to 50 pps
   b. Use at intensities that produce comfortable but visible quadriceps muscle contraction

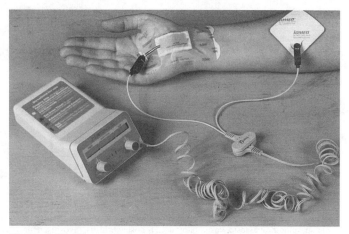

Fig. 25–3. The Transcue II electrode by Empi allows better release of the medications and improved safety than older types of electrodes.

   c. On 8 sec, off 20 sec, with total treatment time of 5–15 min
   d. Discontinue treatment when active muscle contractions restored (usually within 5 sessions)

Contrast Baths

1. Use after acute inflammatory phase
2. Various protocols begin with heat and end with cold; repeat cycle several times
3. Bath temperature and treatment duration depend on level of inflammation
   a. Early subacute phase: warm, short-duration bath followed by relatively long cold treatment
   b. Late subacute phase: hot, longer-lasting initial bath; cooling phase length less crucial

SPINAL INJURIES

Stingers and Burners

1. Immediately ice scalene, trapezius, and levator scapulae muscles to minimize bruising
2. After 72 hr, apply heat: moist heat packs or other modalities
3. ROM and light stretching exercises to recover full, pain-free ROM of cervical spine and involved shoulder
4. Then, slowly progressive strengthening exercise program to build

up stabilizing muscles of neck and scapula; posterior, lateral, and anterior neck muscles; and trapezius and deltoid
5. Continue strengthening exercises during season and offseason

Cervical Disorders

1. Daily strengthening (isometric) and stretching exercises
2. Postural modifications (eg, chin tucks) to control pain
3. When upper extremity radicular pain begins to resolve and pain becomes more axial in trapezius and posterior cervical paraspinal muscles, aggressive exercise, stretching, and postural modifications

Lumbar Disc Herniations

1. Conservative Nonsurgical Therapy
   a. Once radiating leg pain has "centralized," spinal flexor conditioning exercises
   b. Lower extremity stretching and strengthening exercises in low back exercise program, which should last $\geq$ 6 wks
2. Postoperative Rehabilitation
   a. Progress aggressive program incrementally
      (1) Wks 1–2: No strenuous activity
      (2) Wks 3–4: Walk for exercise and perform most activities of daily living
      (3) Wk 4: Begin stationary bike, perhaps stair stepper, and swimming
      (4) Wk 6: Start low back-strengthening exercises and ↑ previous exercises to more strenuous level
      (5) No running until 2–3 mos after surgery
   b. Contact athletes return to sports 6 mos after surgery, though some have returned after only 3 mos

SHOULDER INJURIES

Phases of Rehabilitation

1. Phase I: acute, immediate postinjury or postsurgery phase
   a. Primary goals: to control inflammation and pain, protect damaged or repaired tissue, prevent loss of motion, and minimize loss of strength of injured and surrounding structures
   b. Shoulder positioning controls pain: Resting position is 55° abduction, 30° horizontal adduction, and 0° rotation, with patient in 30–45° recumbency
   c. Exercises (Table 25–2)
      (1) Perform 10–50 reps 2–3 times/day
      (2) Modify if injury aggravated
      (3) Expect few hrs discomfort after exercise, but if 24–48 hrs, modify or discontinue exercise

Table 25–2. Phase I Exercises

Pendulum
Stick or T-bar exercises (passive to active assisted range of motion)
    Flexion
    Abduction in the plane of the scapula (scaption)
    Abduction
    Internal rotation at 0° and 90°
    External rotation at 0° and 90°
Rope and pulley (passive to active assisted range of motion)
    Flexion
    Abduction in the plane of the scapula (scaption)
    Abduction
Active range of motion
    Elbow/wrist/hand
Shoulder isometrics (arm at 0°, elbow at 90°)
    Flexion-extension
    Abduction-adduction
    Internal-external rotation
Scapular retraction and depression

2. Phase II: subacute, strengthening and endurance phase
    a. Primary goals: to regain full passive and active ROM and normal strength of shoulder, and normal aerobic, strength, and endurance level of rest of body
    b. Exercises (Table 25–3)
        (1) General Protocol
            (a) Progress at own rate
            (b) Start with no resistance until proper technique learned
            (c) Then, perform high repetitions and low resistance: 10–50 repetitions 1–2 times/day with 1–3 lb
            (d) With progress to Phase III, cut resistive training back to 2–3 times/wk
        (2) Core exercises for rotator cuff in throwing athletes:
            (a) Prone horizontal abduction (supraspinatus muscle) (Fig. 25-4)
            (b) Prone external rotation at 90° abduction (infraspinatus muscle) (Fig. 25-5)
            (c) Prone extension (teres major) (Fig. 25-6)
        (3) Core exercises for strengthening scapular muscles:
            (a) Pushup plus: normal pushup plus maximum shoulder and scapular protraction with elbows fully extended (serratus anterior)
            (b) Arm elevation in scapular plane in neutral rotation (middle trapezius)
            (c) Press-up (sitting dip): patient sits on table with hands on sides of hips and lifts body off table (pectoralis minor)

Table 25–3. Phase II Exercises

Stretching exercises to obtain terminal range of motion
Stick or T-bar
  Supine external rotation at 135° to 180° abduction
  Side-lying internal rotation at 90° abduction
  Internal rotation pulling the arm up the back
Progressive resistive exercises
  ''Core exercises''
    Prone horizontal abduction (supraspinatus)
    Prone external rotation at 90° abduction (infraspinatus)
    Prone extension (teres minor)
    Pushup plus (serratus anterior)
    Press-up/sitting dips (pectoralis minor)
    Rowing (rhomboids)
    Scaption (trapezius)
  Supplemental shoulder exercises
    Standing
      Flexion
      Abduction
      Internal/external rotation at 0° to 90° with a pulley or rubber tubing
      Diagonal patterns with a pulley or rubber tubing: flexion–abduction–
        external rotation, extension–adduction–internal rotation
    Side-lying external rotation at 0°
    Prone flexion
  Elbow-strengthening exercises
    Biceps curls
    Triceps extensions
    Weight room exercises (modified range of motion not allowing elbows past
      the plane of the shoulder)

       (d) Rowing: pull both arms against resistance toward body
          and pinch shoulder blades together (rhomboids)
  3. Phase III: advanced, sport-specific phase
    a. Started when pain-free, active ROM of shoulder complex is full,
      with minimal (if any) side-to-side difference in manual muscle
      tests of rotator cuff and pericapsular musculature
    b. Primary goals: to prepare shoulder for high-velocity, ballistic
      concentric and eccentric stress and progressively return athlete
      to full sports activity
    c. Focus of Phase III: SAID principle (specific activity to imposed
      demand)
    d. Progressively ↑ concentric and eccentric load capacity of
      shoulder
    e. Exercises
      (1) Oscillatory Motions
        (a) Flexerciser Rod and BodyBlade devices facilitate dy-
          namic co-contraction of shoulder musculature

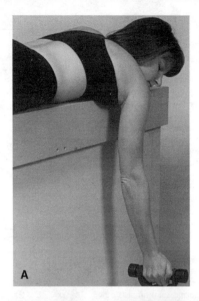

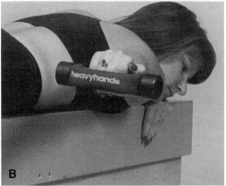

Fig. 25–4. A. Prone horizontal abduction is done with the arm in external rotation, so that the thumb points away from the body. B. The arm is lifted into horizontal abduction until it is parallel to the floor and makes a 90 to 100° angle with the body of the axilla. The arm is held in this position for 3 seconds and then returned to the resting position.

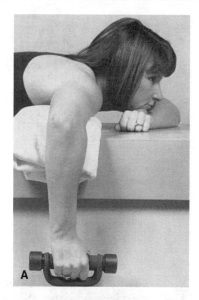

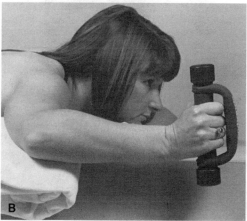

Fig. 25–5. A. Prone external rotation is done with the upper arm supported on the table and the elbow at the edge of the table. B. The forearm is externally rotated until it is parallel with the floor. The arm is held in this position for 3 seconds and then returned to the resting position.

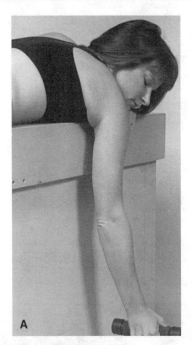

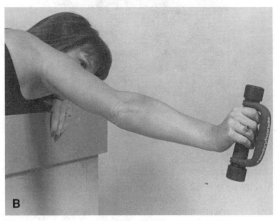

Fig. 25–6. A. Prone extension is done with the arm externally rotated so that the thumb points away from the body. B. The arm is extended until parallel with the floor and held in this position for 3 seconds. The arm is then returned to the resting position.

(b) Arm can be in any position while motions performed

(c) Perform 3–5 sets for 10–30 sec per position or motion

(2) Inertial Exercise

    (a) Impulse device facilitates concentric and eccentric strengthening of musculotendinous unit

    (b) As mass ↓, acceleration forces ↑

    (c) Start with 10–15 lb weight and work toward 1–2 lb, attaining greater acceleration and deceleration speeds to duplicate activity forces

    (d) Perform 1–3 sets of 30 sec per motion

(3) Upper body plyometric training

    (a) Use weighted medicine ball of 2–12 lb

    (b) Progress training from 2-handed to 1-handed activities and simple, pain-free motions to functional, more difficult, and stressful motions

    (c) Focus: quickness of reversing catching to throwing (amortization phase); shorter this phase, > the eccentric stress and concentric force production developed in shoulder musculature

    (d) Perform each motion 3–5 sets of 10–30 reps

Rotator Cuff Tendinitis, Bursitis, and Impingement Syndromes

1. Control acute inflammatory process with relative rest from exacerbating activities for 2 wks, followed by Phase I exercises and pain and inflammation control

2. Once full ROM achieved, perform Phase II strengthening activities for next 4 wks

    a. Modify prone external rotation exercise to side-lying external rotation with arm abducted ≤ 20° until rotator cuff muscles stronger

    b. Activities with arm below 90° elevation usually tolerated better initially, gradually working up to overhead reaching activities

3. Phase III activities started at 6 wks

    a. Goal: to develop eccentric strength of posterior cuff and scapular musculature and posterior cuff flexibility

    b. Passive stretching in internal rotation: patient lies on 1 side with shoulders turned so that affected scapula stabilized against table surface (Fig. 25–7)

4. Postoperative (Debridement and Decompression) Protocol

    a. Start passive and active-assisted ROM and other Phase I exercises 1st day after surgery, and continue for 2–3 wks as tolerated

    b. Phase II: rotator cuff and scapular exercises for 4–6 wks

    c. Add Phase III exercises as soon as athlete has full, pain-free, active ROM and activities

    d. Return to modified or full athletic activities within 8–12 wks

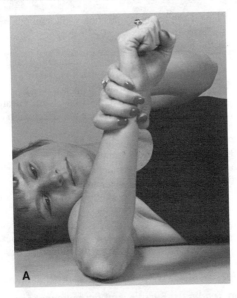

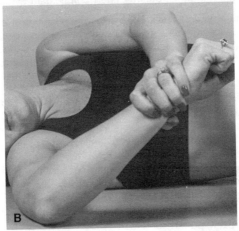

Fig. 25–7. A. Side-lying internal rotation is done with the arm positioned in 90° abduction. B. The patient gently internally rotates the arm with the opposite hand to the point of stretch but not of pain. This position is held for 15 to 20 seconds and the arm then is returned to the starting position.

Rotator Cuff Tears

1. Treat all tears initially with phased rehab for 6–12 wks
2. If normal strength not regained and symptoms recur, surgery needed
3. For partial tears (debridement and decompression), postop rehab same as above, with return to activity in 8–12 wks
4. For complete tears:
   a. Extend Phase I 4–6 wks with passive-assisted exercises (eg, stick and rope and pulley)
   b. Start active-assisted exercises as soon as healing allows, focusing on technique, so substitution patterns not developed
   c. Start Phase II low-resistive isometric or isotonic exercises at 6 wks to restore normal rotator cuff function and strength
   d. Start Phase III activities 4–6 wks later to develop strength
   e. Return to activity: 4–6 mos or longer

Glenoid Labrum Tears

1. Key to conservative treatment: stabilizing glenohumeral joint by enhancing rotator cuff and scapular muscle control
2. Avoid or minimize positions that cause pain or stress
3. Postop rehab after labral debridement (no ligament or labral repair) similar to that after rotator cuff debridement
4. After labral repair, shoulder immobilized for 4–6 wks in internal rotation; thus, important to regain external rotation
5. After SLAP lesion repair, restrict active and resistive elbow flexion exercises and passive shoulder extension exercises for 4–6 wks
6. After repair, Phase I takes 2–4 wks after immobilization, and Phase II and III 6–8 wks each to complete

Glenohumeral Instability

1. Nonsurgical treatment focuses on Phase II and III exercises: dynamic stabilization of glenohumeral joint by rotator cuff and scapular muscles
2. Postop Rehab
   a. Shoulder relatively immobilized for 3–6 wks
   b. Start isometric shoulder exercises within 2–3 wks
   c. Start Phase I active-assisted ROM exercises after immobilization so shoulder muscles protect repaired capsular tissue
   d. Frequently, gradual return of external rotation and elevation ROM extended over 3-month period
   e. Start Phase II exercises 2–4 wks after immobilization; early incorporation of scapular stabilization exercises and normal scapulohumeral patterns lessens chance of poor biomechanical motions developing
   f. Add Phase III exercises 3–4 mos postop and practice for 3–4 mos

Proximal Humerus Fractures

1. Start passive-assisted exercises early when fracture or fracture repair stable
2. With minimally displaced fracture, start ROM exercises within 7–10 days if tolerated
3. Warm-up with heat to affected area, followed by stretching
4. Early rehab: assisted elbow flexion and extension, pendulum exercises, and supine lateral rotation.
5. As strength ↑, exercise 3–4 times/day to ensure full restoration of abduction and external and internal rotation
6. Start isometric exercises at 3–4 wks
7. Use light weights as early as 12 wks
8. If pain excessive during exercise or weight lifting, ↓ or discontinue weight lifting

ELBOW INJURIES

Lateral Epicondylitis

1. Primary goals: to reduce pain and tenderness, and restore strength, endurance, and flexibility of wrist extensors at elbow
2. Counterforce bracing of extensor carpi radialis brevis
   a. Creates pressure over muscle bellies and dissipates impact load through muscles, taking stress off inflamed tendons
   b. Wear brace 1 inch distal to elbow so full flexion possible
   c. Wear brace at all times, except when sleeping or bathing
3. During acute stage, wear brace, exercise without weights, and rest elbow
4. Once acute symptoms subside, start stretching and strengthening exercises
   a. "Super 7" exercises: grip strengthening, stretching extensors (Fig. 25–8), wrist curls (Fig. 25–9), reverse curls, neutral wrist curls, pronation, and supination (Fig. 25–10)
   b. Perform deep friction massage 3 times/day for 3–5 mins
5. Use therapeutic modalities: moist heat before exercise, ice after exercise, iontophoresis, phonophoresis, galvanic stimulation
6. Return to activity: 2–3 wks
7. Stretch before and after competition and ice after activity
8. If surgery needed, immobilize extremity in long-arm splint at 90° flexion for 1 wk, then start gentle stretch exercises and active wrist ROM
   a. Start active elbow ROM exercises after 2–3 wks
   b. Start stretching and strengthening exercises at 3–4 wks
   c. Continue exercises until full strength returns (within 4–5 mos)

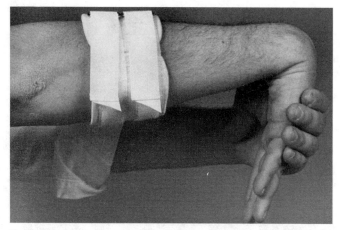

Fig. 25–8. Stretching the extensors is done with the arm held out in front, palm facing the ground, and the elbow extended. The patient uses the unaffected hand to pull the hand of the affected side so that the wrist flexes.

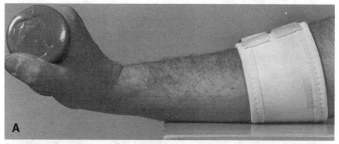

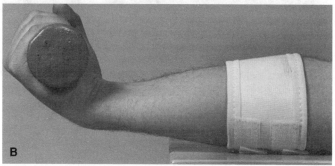

Fig. 25–9. Wrist curls are done with the forearm supported, leaving the wrist free to have full motion. (A) Flexors; (B) Extensors.

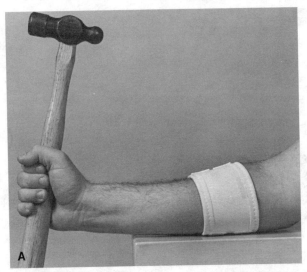

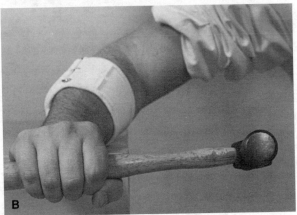

Fig. 25–10. (A) Neutral wrist curls, (B) pronation, and (C) supination.

    d. Return to athletic activity possible within 6 wks if sport technique modified

Simple Dislocations

1. After reduction, place arm in posterior long-arm splint with elbow flexed 90° and forearm fully pronated for 2–3 days
2. ROM Exercises

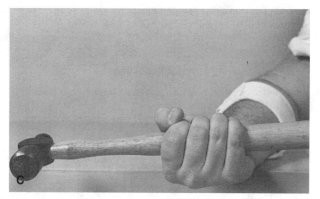

Fig. 25–10. *(continued).*

    a. Avoid early passive ROM exercises, as they exacerbate tissue trauma and may result in heterotopic ossification

    b. Start active ROM exercises in pain-free range in anti-gravity position; by 2 wks, range should approach 80–100° arc

    c. No limit on flexion; limit extension initially only if instability at terminal extension

    d. If motion restoration slower than expected, start active-assisted exercises after 2 wks

    e. Reduce edema by ICE and electrogalvanic stimulation to help restore early motion

3. If elbow stable, discontinue splint in 1–2 wks; if not, splint for 4 wks, adjusting for more extension as tolerated and as stability permits; if, at 4–6 wks, flexion contracture still evident, extension orthosis can help restore full extension

4. Use laterally or medially hinged splint that allows free motion in protected range; wear for 4 wks and then remove for full motion, but use for support during activities

5. Start isometric exercises

6. Start strengthening program after full, active ROM achieved (within 6–8 wks)

    a. Exercises: wrist curls, supination and pronation, biceps and triceps curls, and grip strengthening

    b. If extension loss, focus on strengthening triceps to resist elbow flexion during forced extension activities

7. Delay elbow loading until strength restored and ROM within 30° of preinjury capability (usually 2–3 mos)

8. If signs of heterotopic calcification, stop all strengthening exercises and continue only active ROM

9. Use Scotchwrap (3M) to splint elbow for return to play: prevents hyperextension, but allows full ROM
10. Unrestricted return to play when ROM is full, pain-free, and stable (within 3–6 mos)

Dislocations Requiring Surgical Reduction

1. Immobilize elbow in long-arm cast at 90° flexion with forearm fully pronated
   a. Wear cast for 4 wks, then hinged cast with extension block of 30° for 6 wks
   b. Remove extension block if no evidence of ligamentous laxity; younger patients or those with generalized laxity may need extension block splint for up to 6 mos
2. Continue splint for ≥ 3 mos postop, after which ROM exercises allowed in forearm rotation
3. No loaded activities for ≥ 6 mos postop, and no extension past neutral

Medial Epicondyle Fractures

1. Nondisplaced or Minimally Displaced Fractures
   a. Initially, immobilize with posterior splint
   b. Start active-assisted ROM exercises 4–5 days after injury
   c. Discard splint when swelling and tenderness minimal
   d. Return to activity when ROM and strength full
2. Postop Rehab
   a. Start ROM exercises as soon as tolerated (as early as 1 wk)
   b. Remove splint 3 wks after surgery
   c. Start strengthening exercises when ROM full
   d. Return to progressive throwing within 6–8 wks

Type I Coronoid Fractures

1. Immobilize elbow for 3–4 days, then start ROM exercises
2. Therapy progression and activity return dictated by symptoms
3. No protection needed during competition

Nondisplaced Radial Head Fractures

1. Place arm in sling for 2–3 days, then start flexion and extension exercises, adding pronation and supination later
2. Resume activities of daily living as tolerated
3. Moist heat to elbow before exercise relaxes tissues and promotes better active ROM
4. Complete exercises actively in anti-gravity position or with constant passive motion (CPM) machine
5. Attain full ROM early to prevent adverse effects on throwing of lack of full extension

6. Unrestricted return to activity when ROM full and painless (usually 2–3 mos)

7. No protective equipment needed, but hinged elbow support may be helpful

Sprains

1. Initial treatment: ice and continue normal ROM

2. When ROM normal, start progressive resistance exercises

3. Gradual return to play; tape to protect against hyperextension and medial stresses

Contusions

1. Treat with rest and ice

2. Treat bursitis with several days' compression and avoid exacerbating activities

3. Treat myositis ossificans by protecting injured arm and starting early active ROM

WRIST AND HAND INJURIES

Fractures of the Distal Radius

1. After cast removed, start active and passive wrist and digit ROM exercises

2. Warm wrist joint for 15–20 mins before exercise

3. Therapeutic modalities: fluidotherapy, hydrocollators, paraffin

4. Once ROM achieved, start strengthening exercises

5. Return to play within 6–8 wks, but use playing splint and continue ROM and strengthening exercises

Scaphoid Fractures

1. After casting or surgery, start active ROM and therapeutic modalities

2. Start resistive exercises within 2 mos

3. Return to play only after adequate healing (2–6 wks) and wearing protective splint

Metacarpal Fractures

1. Usually casted, but Galveston Metacarpal Brace (Fig. 25–11) may be used for metacarpals 2–4

    a. 3-point pressure fracture reduction allows motion at wrist, MCP, and IP joints

    b. Place larger pad on dorsum transversely over apex of fracture, and align crossbar with 2 smaller pads with long axis of fractured metacarpal, 1 pad proximal and 1 pad distal to fracture

    c. Monitor pressure on closure with dorsal pad; 2 colors of dorsal

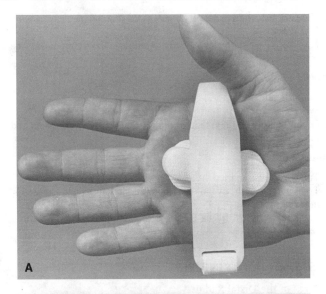

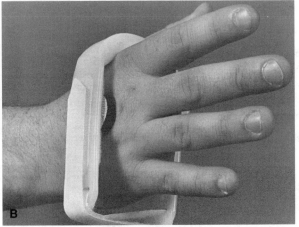

Fig. 25-11. The Galveston Metacarpal Brace to reduce metacarpal fractures. (A) Volar view. (B) Dorsal view.

pad must be visible after reduction and pressure must be comfortable to athlete

2. Return to play with protective playing splint as symptoms permit

Mallet Finger

1. Splint with DIP joint extended and other joints free for 6–9 wks joint before starting active flexion exercises
2. Continue splint up to 12 wks if DIP cannot actively extend
3. Continue playing after injury using splint

Avulsions of the Flexor Digitorum Profundus

1. After surgery, wear dorsal splint for 3 wks with wrist slightly flexed, MCP joint flexed 60–70°, and IP joints extended
2. After 3 wks, perform active ROM exercises (blocking and composite) throughout day
3. Until 5th wk, perform all exercises in protected position and take splint off only for exercises
4. Initiate light activities of daily living when splint discontinued; start more strenuous exercises at 8 wks
5. Return to play within 3 wks using protective silicone playing splint, continuing protection until mobility full

Articular Fractures of the PIP Joint

1. Start rehab well before fracture completely healed
2. Remove splint 2–3 wks after injury or surgery, and protectively exercise finger several times/day
3. At 4 wks, start passive mobilization
4. Protective splint and buddy taping may allow early return to sports activity

Fracture-Dislocations of the PIP Joint

1. After surgery, splint finger at 25° flexion for 2–3 wks, then start gentle active exercises
2. No full extension until 4 wks after surgery; during interim, may use extension block splint

Boutonnière Deformity

1. Splint PIP joint in extension for at least 6–8 wks, with DIP joint free to actively flex and extend
2. After 6–8 wks, start active ROM, wearing splint at night
3. Continue buddy taping (assists in active ROM) as long as joint sore
4. May compete if digit protected

Dislocations of the PIP Joint

1. Dorsal Dislocations
   a. Reduce, then splint digit at 30° flexion (to prevent full extension) for 3–4 wks

    b. For return to play, protect injured digit with buddy taping and padded splint
2. Volar Dislocations
    a. Repair surgically and splint PIP joint at 0° extension for 6 wks
    b. Return to play as symptoms permit, keeping digit splinted

"Gamekeeper's" or "Skier's" Thumb

1. Immobilize thumb in 20° flexion with IP joint free for active motion and to prevent extensor mechanism scarring
2. Grade I Injury: splint immobilization for 3 wks, followed by active and passive ROM, edema control, and cryotherapy
3. Grade II Injury: splint immobilization for 5 wks (hand-based thumb spica prevents ulnar and radial deviation of joint), followed by rehab exercises, with return to play in 1–2 wks if nondominant hand and 4–6 wks if dominant hand
    a. If surgery needed, wear cast for 4 wks postop, followed by active and passive ROM, edema control, and taping to ↓ stiffness
    b. Start strengthening exercises at 6 wks
    c. Return to play 2–9 wks after surgery if thumb protected, either by buddy taping in adduction to index finger or silicone splint

Wrist and Hand Splints for Return to Competition

1. Specialized splints to prevent re-injury: lightweight, compact, and cause minimal interference
2. For athletic competition, below-elbow splints cannot be made from unyielding material
3. GE RTV-11 Silicone Splint: application similar to thinly "icing" cake
4. 3M Scotchwrap Splint: less rigid fiberglass splint applied like fiberglass cast

MUSCULOTENDINOUS INJURIES ABOUT THE KNEE

Hamstring Strain

1. Rehab starts with isometric exercises: contract hamstrings without moving hip or knee joint
    a. Perform exercises with knee joint at various angles within pain-free range
    b. Change knee angle in 20° increments
2. Start isotonic exercises when isometric exercises are pain free
    a. Do prone, flexing knee against gravity
    b. Initially, only leg weight used for 1–2 sets of 10 repetitions
    c. Isotonics ↑, isometrics ↓ and are discontinued
        (1) ↑ sets of 10 repetitions until performing 3 sets/session, ≤ 3 times/day

(2) With pain as guide, ↑ weight in 2–3 lb increments no more often than every 2 days

(3) Each time weight ↑, ↓ and then gradually ↑ number of sets as pain permits

(4) When lifting 15 lbs for 3 sets of 10 reps 3 times/day, start isokinetics

3. Isokinetic exercises performed on Biodex-type machine (controls speed of motion)

   a. Performed in concentric (muscle-shortening) contraction mode

   b. Start at 240°/sec for 3 sets of 10 reps

   c. Then ↑ speed to 300°/sec for 2 sets of 30

   d. As progress allows, ↓ speed and add 3 sets of 10 reps

   e. If isokinetic equipment not available, walk or run backward

   f. Once concentric training performed without difficulty, start eccentric (muscle-lengthening) contraction exercises

   g. With eccentric work, start speed at 30°/sec and advance to faster speeds

   h. Forward running useful for eccentric training of hamstrings

Quadriceps Strains

1. 1st isotonic exercises: straight leg raises
2. Perform other exercises seated, with thigh resting on treatment table and heel resting on variable height stool to keep knee within pain-free range

   a. Perform terminal knee extensions

   b. ↑ weight up to 20 lbs in 2–3 lb increments, no more often than every 2 days

   c. Perform quadriceps isometric and isotonic exercises and progress to hamstring exercises

3. Isokinetic exercises performed similar to hamstring exercises, but concentric training like forward running and eccentric training like backward running
4. Carefully stretch quadriceps in prone position to prevent further injury
5. Start general conditioning program 2–3 days after injury, but no biking until active knee motion is 100°

Return to Sports After Muscle Strains

1. Equal flexibility and endurance
2. Function on isokinetic testing within 10% of noninjured extremity
3. If no isokinetic equipment, test function: if no discomfort with sprinting 50 yds 3 times and running 3 15-yd figure-of-eights at full speed, return to competition

Quadriceps Contusions

1. Initial Phase: restore knee motion, guided by daily knee pain and ROM evaluation

    a. Weight bearing as tolerated, and discontinue crutches when motion $> 90°$

    b. Never use heat: it ↑ risk of rebleeding

    c. Continue ice massage when performing flexion-extension gravity-assisted motion

    d. Continue treatment until pain-free active knee flexion $> 120°$

2. Progress to functional rehab and return to competition

    a. Perform sport-specific activities and agility drills (eg, running, cutting, jumping) with ↑ speed

    b. With full ROM of knee and successful completion of functional tests, return to competition if thigh adequately protected

Acute Compartment Syndromes of the Thigh

1. Postop rehab varies with fasciotomy wound size and amount of necrosis

    a. Start passive ROM and partial weight-bearing exercises immediately postop to reduce edema

    b. As wound heals and weight bearing ↑, start progressive resistance training

2. Add ROM, strengthening, and light jogging as tolerated until starting functional activities

3. Return to sports activity within 8–12 wks with thigh protection

EXTENSOR MECHANISM (EM) INJURIES

Significance of Vastus Medialis Obliquus (VMO) Strengthening

1. VMO provides dynamic medial pull to align patella in femoral groove

2. With EM dysfunction, rehab trains VMO in most optimal position, encouraging firing before vastus lateralis for proper patellar positioning

3. Exercises for selective VMO strengthening

    a. Straight leg raises with external twisting

    b. Simultaneous bilateral heel lifts while squeezing rubber ball or pillow between distal thighs to create hip adduction

    c. Side-lying hip adduction with VMO maintaining anti-gravity position

Exercises for EM Injuries

1. Flexibility Exercises

    a. Hamstring flexibility extremely important: stretch if any tightness

    b. Stretch gastrocnemius-soleus group, quadriceps, and iliotibial band

2. Balancing exercises performed on devices that improve proprioceptive function also enhance agility and coordination

3. When strengthening, flexibility, and coordination attained, progressive running program returns athlete to activity
   a. Brisk walking, then alternating straight-ahead walking and jogging, then running straight ahead for ↑ distances
   b. Depending on sport, follow with shorter-distance sprinting and cutting with various techniques in different directions

Types of Exercises

1. Start isometric exercise (ie, quadriceps sets [Fig. 25–12] and straight leg raises) during initial stages EM dysfunction
2. Isolate quadriceps (eg, have patient sit): if knee painful, easier to contract using hamstrings and hip extensors
3. Flexion-to-extension exercise (open chain: proximal segment fixed and distal segment moves) causes both concentric shortening and eccentric lengthening of muscle fibers
4. Closed-chain exercise (fixed foot, proximal segment moves) is more functional
5. Isokinetic exercises: athlete works at high speeds against varying resistance (closed-chain method) to avoid further irritation
6. Effect on patellofemoral joint reaction force (PFJRF): ↑ compression force between patella and femur as knee flexed
   a. Open-chain exercises ↑ PFJRF, which may further irritate joint by applying compressive loads to patella
   b. Closed-chain exercises also ↑ PFJRF, but disperse patellofemoral forces more evenly
   c. Isokinetic exercises ↓ PFJRF and closely mimic quadriceps activities during sports
7. Combine isometric, concentric, and eccentric components in weight-bearing exercises
   a. Progress from isometrics standing to functional exercises (step-ups, squats, lunges, slide board [Fig. 25–13]) and other sport-mimicking activities
   b. Closed-chain exercises heavily emphasize pelvis, knee, and foot control, improving proprioception and kinesthetic awareness

Anterior Knee Pain

1. Goals: to gain optimal patellar position by taping and stretching tight soft tissue components and then functionally improving VMO firing pattern
2. Progress rehab from correcting patellar position with McConnell taping (Fig. 25–14) to improving lower extremity mechanics and control in sport activity
   a. Correcting abnormal patellar position allows for optimal VMO function and pain-free exercising
   b. Begin exercises in nonweight-bearing position, progressing to weight bearing, closed-chain exercises (eg, stance quadriceps

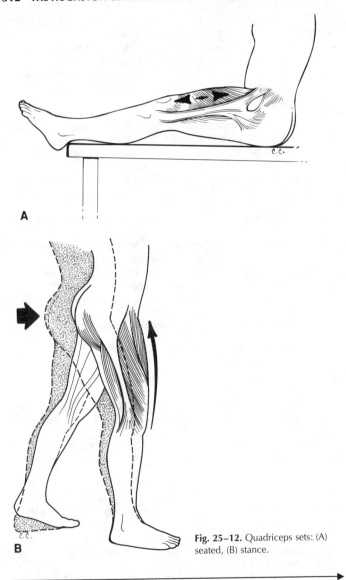

Fig. 25–12. Quadriceps sets: (A) seated, (B) stance.

Fig. 25–13. Athletes progress to functional exercises that mimic motions used in sports, such as the slide board (A) and marching against resistance (B).

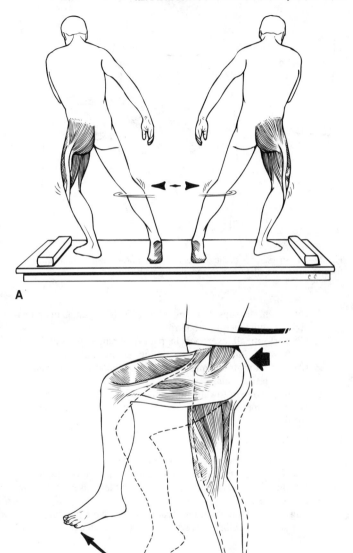

A

B

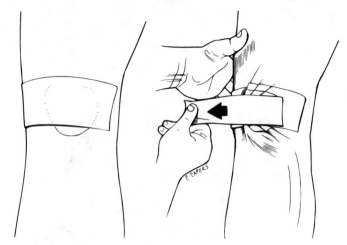

Fig. 25–14. An example of the McConnell taping program in which taping is used to correct patellar position and allow pain-free exercise.

activation, step-ups, step-downs, and 10–15° squats), all emphasizing pelvis-knee-foot control

   (1) Perform all exercises in pain-free range, progressing as VMO firing and lower extremity control improve

   (2) Stretch gastrocnemius, hamstrings, iliotibial band, and lateral retinaculum

  c. Then gear rehab toward functional training in sport, gradually weaning from taping as VMO firing improves and symptoms subside

Plica Irritation

1. Treat synovial irritation and proliferation by ↓ swelling
2. Emphasize ↑ hamstrings flexibility and quadriceps strengthening with isometrics, quadriceps sets, and straight leg raises; flexion-to-extension exercises aggravate synovial lining
3. Taping may worsen irritation because of excessive pressure
4. Once pain and swelling resolve, progress to rehab exercises that ↑ PFJRF

Patellar Instability

1. Treat acute subluxation with RICE and isometric exercises
2. Knee sleeve or lateral felt pad with Ace wrap supports for 3–5 days, allowing medial tissues to heal
3. Start electrical stimulation, biofeedback, and McConnell taping as soon as possible to promote VMO activation

Patellar Dislocation

1. Rehab aimed at ↓ effusion, allowing medial retinaculum to heal in taut position and activating quadriceps
   a. Compressive dressing with felt, lateral, C-shaped pad, and knee immobilizer
   b. Perform active ankle pumps, quadriceps sets with VMO emphasis, and straight leg raises in immobilizer
   c. Cryotherapy and electrical stimulation reduce swelling
2. Crutches and touch-down weight bearing for 2–3 wks
3. Remove splint after 2–3 wks and fit with neoprene sleeve or McConnell taping if tolerable
4. Progress from no weight bearing to closed-chain exercises as tolerated
5. Flexion exercises: sit with legs over table end and use active resistive flexion against therapist's hand
   a. Quadriceps reflexively relaxed, allowing hamstrings to flex knee
   b. Perform flexion 3–4 times/day for 5–7 mins to prevent swelling
6. When not doing flexion exercises, keep knee extended to promote medial retinaculum healing in shortened position
7. Wean off crutches as quadriceps control in weight bearing improves
   a. McConnell taping beneficial as swelling ↓ and athlete progresses toward functional activities
   b. External tape support provides security and proprioception to VMO during closed-chain exercises

Patellar Tendinitis ("Jumper's" Knee)

1. Initial treatment: rest from activity; ice, heat, deep massage, and iontophoresis; flexibility program for hamstrings, quadriceps, and heel cords
2. Follow with isometric quadriceps-strengthening program: start in full extension and progress to flexion with weight-bearing closed-chain exercises
3. Then isotonic exercises to strengthen hamstrings, quadriceps, and hip muscles (ROM of each exercise must be completely painless)
4. Eccentric exercises using isokinetics to progressively strengthen tensile components of patellar tendon beneficial
   a. Closed-chain exercises encompass eccentric action of quadriceps, causing less PFJRF
   b. Quick stretch, 15–20° single knee squats, side step-ups, and forward lunges ↑ quadriceps eccentric strength
5. During early rehab, jumping athlete starts with slow movement (eg, cycling, jogging, straight-leg hip flexion and extension) in deep water with flotation device, then progresses to more difficult exercises in shallow water
6. "Drop and stop" technique also beneficial
   a. After warm-up and quadriceps and hamstrings stretching (static or proprioceptive neuromuscular facilitation) , ↑ semisquat exer-

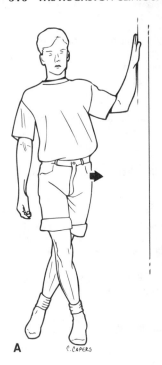

A

C. CAPERS

Fig. 25–15. (A) Stretching exercise for the (left) iliotibial band in the standing position. (B) Stretching exercise for the (left) iliotibial band using the opposite foot to assist stabilization and maximize the stretch. (C) Stretching exercise for the (left) iliotibial band; the patient may rotate at the waist away from the affected side.

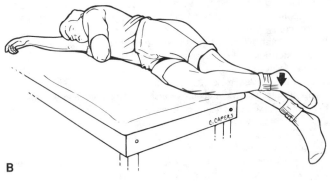

B

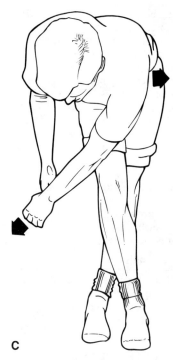

C

Fig. 25–15. *(continued).*

cises, starting with larger and faster squats and progressing to
weights
b. Conclude session with recovery exercises (stretching) and local
ice
7. Pain free before return to sport; may wear knee sleeve or infrapatellar band

Osgood-Schlatter Disease

1. After acute stage, quadriceps and hamstrings stretching and
strengthening exercises, isometric contractions 1st, then isotonics
2. Start concentric exercises in 2nd phase
3. Last phase of rehab: eccentric exercises

Iliotibial Band Syndrome

1. Stretching exercises for iliotibial band, tensor fascia lata, external
rotator muscles of hip, and hamstrings (Fig. 25–15) continued
throughout program

2. Proprioceptive neuromuscular facilitation (PNF) stretching techniques in advanced phase, when brace discontinued
3. No running until lateral femoral epicondyle pain disappears; if lateral pain returns, discontinue running
4. Correct predisposing factors
   a. Endurance runners may need to reduce mileage
   b. Short-track or banked-road runners should run on different surfaces or change frequently road side and direction run
   c. Wear suitable running shoes
   d. Special orthoses to control excessive valgus foot pronation or genu varum and lower extremity asymmetry

Popliteus Tendinitis

1. Stretching and strengthening quadriceps, hamstrings, and popliteus exercises
2. Correct training errors
3. Progressive normalization of training session, leaving downhill work for final phase

Biceps Femoris Tendinitis

1. Rest from activity, local ice, and functional knee taping
2. Progress from adequate stretching cycle (including PNF techniques) and hamstrings strengthening exercises through isometric and isotonic exercises, and finally eccentric exercises

LIGAMENTOUS KNEE INJURIES

General Guidelines

1. ROM
   a. After extra-articular surgery, immobilize knee in 45–60° flexion for 4–6 wks
      (1) After immobilization, only active and gradual ROM into extension: gaining 5°/wk acceptable
      (2) Final 5° flexion contracture acceptable
      (3) Only after 12–14 wks use passive motion to gain extension
      (4) Start flexion activities passively and aggressively when cast removed, with goal of full flexion by 12 wks
   b. After intra-articular surgery, passive ROM exercises stress graft initially to maintain full extension
      (1) Perform with ankle or heel propped on pillow or bolster (Fig. 25–16) or lying prone with leg extended off table and knee supported
      (2) Regain full extension by 3–4 wks
      (3) Start flexion activities day after surgery; attain 90° flexion within 4–5 days and full flexion within 4–6 wks

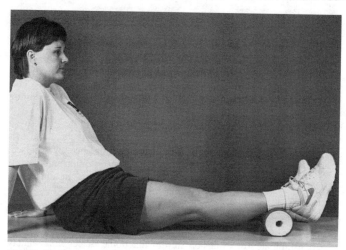

Fig. 25–16. Passive extension is gained by having the patient prop the ankle or heel on a pillow or bolster or lie prone extending the leg off the table with the knee supported.

2. Continuous Passive Motion (CPM)
   a. No CPM after extra-articular surgery
   b. After intra-articular surgery, start active and passive ROM exercises and weight bearing immediately; thus, CPM not needed for most patients
   c. CPM shortcomings
      (1) Device axis cannot follow knee through full ROM
      (2) May apply inappropriate forces
3. Gait and Weight Bearing
   a. Start normal gait weight bearing as soon as possible
   b. Altered gait pattern only if knee must be held in limited motion (eg, after acute injury or extra-articular surgery)
      (1) Rather than landing on heel with knee extended, bear weight on ball of foot
      (2) To use crutches, place ball of foot down, contract knee muscles to stabilize knee, and step through
      (3) Once ROM and strength improved and ligament protection phase ended, attempt normal heel-toe gait
   c. After intra-articular surgery, attempt normal heel-toe gait as soon as possible
4. Muscle Strengthening
   a. Perform high-repetition, low-weight exercises after immobilization during healing phase

   b. Initial regimen: 5–10 sets of 10 reps, 2–3 times/day, using ≤ 10 lbs
   c. Hip musculature and hamstrings: 5 sets of 10 reps, 1–2 times/ day
   d. Quadriceps: 2–3 times/day with more repetitions; take knee to fullest possible extension with leg lifts
   e. Start closed-chain activities slowly with 10–50 reps, depending on activity
5. Proprioception
   a. To improve balance and kinesthetic awareness: stand and balance on 1 leg, rise up on ball of foot and balance, eyes closed
   b. Equipment available to train and test proprioception and balance
   c. Significant knee proprioception provided by its muscular support, so muscles focus of much rehab
6. Bracing
   a. Select postop braces for accurate ROM adjustments and allowing flexion and extension stops as necessary
   b. Eliminate 10° extension stop in functional braces immediately postop to discourage flexion contractures
   c. Reactivate stop once athlete ready to engage in vigorous activities
   d. 10° stop beneficial in controlling unreconstructed knees

Nonsurgically Treated Medial Compartment Injuries

1. Heal best with controlled ROM
   a. Hinged immobilizer prevents last 20° extension, providing protected weight bearing and preventing capsular stress
   b. Allow full flexion
   c. Protected weight bearing with crutches for ≥ 3 wks
2. Start quadriceps sets, terminal knee extensions, straight leg raises, hamstrings curls, and exercises for hip flexors, abductors, and extensors immediately
   a. Use high reps with light weights
   b. Start bicycling as soon as tolerated
3. Progress from partial to full weight bearing and out of immobilizer (may take 4–6 wks)
4. Once bearing full weight, start closed-chain exercises
5. Start isotonic and isokinetic exercises once ligaments are healing
6. Progress through functional exercise continuum until able to pass functional testing and return to full activity

Surgically Treated Medial Compartment Injuries

1. Emphasis on early motion to restore optimal ligament strength
2. Protect knee during mobilization to avoid disruption of repaired structures and allow healing
   a. Protect with cast brace or rehab brace (Fig. 25–17)

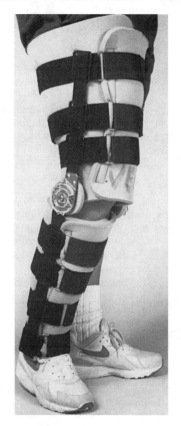

Fig. 25-17. A hinged immobilizer is used after surgery to prevent unwanted extension and flexion while allowing motion within the permissible range.

    b. Rehab braces usually have Velcro or adjustable straps to allow circumferential size changes to allow for swelling postop

    c. Longitudinal medial and lateral struts protect against valgus stress

    d. Adjustable hinges protect knee against extremes of motion while allowing ''safe range'' mobilization

  3. Initially restrict terminal extension to avoid posteromedial corner stress

Specific Medial Ligament Complex Sprains

  1. Grade I Sprains

    a. Protected weight bearing with crutches

    b. Start isometric exercises immediately, rapidly progressing to resistive exercises

    c. As discomfort ↓, discontinue crutches and start mobilization

    d. More aggressive program to restore strength, endurance, flexibility, and ROM

2. Grade II Sprains

    a. Rehab brace that allows full motion, but protects against valgus stress usually more comfortable

    b. Protected weight bearing with crutches

    c. Start isometric exercises immediately, rapidly advancing to progressive resistive exercises as tolerated

    d. As discomfort diminishes and stability returns, discontinue crutches and brace

3. Grade III Sprains

    a. Hold postop lower extremity in limited-motion brace, restricting last 30° extension

    b. Some recommend early protected motion from 0–90°

    c. Brace protection and crutch ambulation for 6 wks after surgery

    d. Isometric exercises and leg raises, rapidly advancing to progressive resistive exercises during protection period

    e. After protection period, restore full ROM with active and passive modalities

    f. Progressive weight bearing as stability, motion, and strength return

    g. Enhance muscle strength, flexibility, and endurance with aggressive, early, closed-chain exercises

    h. Functional strengthening, sport-specific exercises, and agility drills, with return to sport dictated by return of motion, flexibility, strength, and endurance

Acute ACL Injury with ALRI

1. If partially torn ACL needs protection, use only very light resistance for quadriceps work; limit heavier quadriceps exercises from 90–45° to decrease anterior translation forces associated with full-arc extensions

2. Hinged immobilizer at 20° protects capsular ligaments

3. Control weight bearing with crutches and 3-point gait pattern, progressing weight bearing as tolerated; discontinue crutches when ambulating comfortably without limp

4. Quadriceps sets, terminal knee extensions, straight leg raises, hamstrings curls, and strengthening of hip abductors, adductors, and extensors

    a. Attain initial flexion gains by sitting with thigh supported on bench and feet off floor (Fig. 25–18); use uninjured leg to provide active-assisted motion

    b. Lying prone with leg suspended over table edge allows easier knee extension (Fig. 25–19)

5. Progress from general closed-chain exercise (eg, minimal squats,

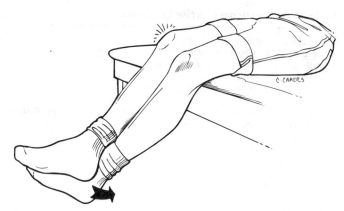

Fig. 25–18. Sitting position used to help regain initial flexion. The uninjured leg is used to provide active assisted support. Generally, the patient is able to relax in this position and to regain flexion more rapidly.

cycling, rubber tubing squats, and light leg presses) to more vigorous exercises (eg, half squats, heavier leg presses, stair climber)
6. Depending on healing (regaining full extension, flexion near normal, effusion resolved, hamstrings strength $\geq$ 90%, quadriceps strength $\geq$ 70%), may progress to more functional activities (Tables 25–4 and 25–5) within 4–6 wks, wearing functional brace

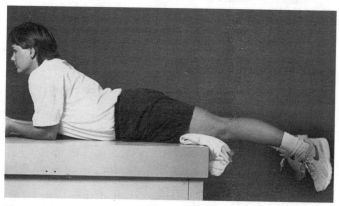

Fig. 25–19. Prone position for regaining extension. This position again allows for more complete relaxation.

Table 25–4. Functional Exercise Continuum

Closed-chain continuum
   Leg press with rubber tubing and progress to machines
   Wall slides or mini-squat, mini-trampoline
   One-leg sissy squat
   Tubing squats, two legs progressing to one
   Step-ups and side step-ups
   Hops against tubing side to side, two legs, one leg, one leg agility, plyometrics
Ambulation continuum
   No weight bearing
   Partial weight bearing
   Walk 2 miles
   Stride/jog 2 miles
   Sprint 40 yards
   Cutting
   Deceleration
   Sport specific
Functional testing
   General hop test: one jump, three jumps, timed, and side to side
   Figure-of-eight run
   Sprint speed
   Endurance run
   Agility run: T test
   Proprioceptive testing
   Carioca
   Isokinetic testing

7. Interval running program: straight-ahead jogging, then ↑ speeds, and finally agility exercises
8. Add balancing drills to improve proprioception, add sport-specific drills, and continue strengthening exercises
9. Return to sport when hamstrings strength equal to uninjured leg and quadriceps strength ≥ 80% normal

Surgically Treated AMRI

1. Initially lock knee from 45–60° (some say full extension) in hinged immobilizer
   a. Quadriceps and hamstrings sets, straight leg raises, and strengthening of hip abductors, adductors, and extensors
   b. Toe-touch weight bearing with crutches
   c. In acute injury, open immobilizer hinge from 30–70°
2. Discontinue immobilizer at 6 wks and start general active ROM and muscle strengthening
   a. Gain extension through active motion, flexion through active and passive motion

Table 25–5. Rehabilitation Protocol for Patients with Acute Nonoperatively Treated Rotatory Instability (AMRI, ALRI)*

Phase	Activities
Immobilization	Hinged brace allowing 20° to full extension for 3 to 6 weeks, depending on ligament laxity tests
Ambulation	Two-crutch touch-down weight bearing
	One-crutch as quadriceps improves
	Full weight bearing once brace use is ended
	Begin running in brace as tolerated
	Full range of motion when out of brace
Exercise	Strength exercises at 5 to 10 sets a day using no more than 10-pound weights
	Quadriceps sets
	Terminal knee extensions
	Straight leg raises with terminal knee extensions
	Hip flexion
	Hip extension
	Hip adduction
	Hip abduction
	Hamstrings curls
Functional progression	Weight room and aggressive closed-chain activities

* Key: AMRI, anteromedial rotatory instability: ALRI, anterolateral rotatory instability.

    b. Perform closed-chain exercises: quadriceps sets, terminal knee extensions, straight leg raises, and exercises for hip flexors, adductors, abductors, and extensors
      (1) Start progressive resistive exercises within 1st few wks using light weights ($\leq$ 5 lbs) as tolerated
      (2) Perform hamstring-resisted exercises throughout full ROM and quadriceps exercises in limited arc (90–60°)
    c. Partial weight bearing at 6 wks, progressing to full weight bearing as knee extension and quadriceps control improve (within 10–12 wks)
  3. Upon restoration of ROM, adequate muscle control and strength, and resolution of effusion, progress to functional rehab, then more strenuous isotonic and isokinetic exercises as tolerated
  4. Full return to activity once functional guidelines satisfactorily met
    a. Functional brace effective in resisting varus and valgus loads and hyperextension
    b. Use brace during sports for 1st yr postop; base further use on patient preference

Surgically Treated AL-AMRI

1. Extra-Articular Surgery (Table 25–6)
   a. Lock knee in hinged immobilizer at 45°
   b. Acutely injured athlete may have limited ROM from 30–70° after 3 wks
   c. Immobilize chronic injury for 6 wks
      (1) Touch-down weight bearing only for 6 wks, then gradually ↑ weight bearing
      (2) Remove immobilizer at 6 wks, though may use during sleep to prevent passive extension
   d. ↑ ROM using active exercises for extension and passive motion for flexion
   e. Up to time of full weight bearing, perform quadriceps sets, terminal knee extensions, straight leg raises, and strengthening of hip adductors, abductors, and extensors
   f. Once weight bearing with crutches comfortable, start closed-chain exercises
   g. While progressing through functional exercise continuum, work toward returning to sport-specific activities (takes 6–8 mos)
2. Intra-Articular Surgery (Table 25–7)
   a. Requires full extension from postoperative day 1
      (1) Hold knee in full-extension immobilizer
      (2) Touch-down weight bearing as tolerated
      (3) Take immobilizer off for passive extension and active-assisted flexion exercises 1st day after surgery
      (4) Start quadriceps sets, terminal knee extensions (assisted with electrical stimulation and biofeedback), and straight leg raises
   b. Encourage flexion to 90° within 5–7 days, progressing motion as tolerated over next 7–10 days
   c. Continue quadriceps sets, terminal knee extensions, straight leg raises, hip flexors, hamstrings curls, aggressive knee flexion, and minimum standing knee bends after discharge; start other hip exercises as soon as tolerated
   d. Discontinue immobilizer once gait normal
   e. Use crutches until quadriceps strength appropriate and gait steady
   f. Start cycling as soon as wounds heal and ROM is sufficient
   g. Use light resistance with exercises, with goal of 10 lbs by 6–10 wks
   h. Avoid high-resistance, isokinetic, and isotonic open-chain extension exercises for 4–6 mos
   i. Full return to activity usually within 6–7 mos

Table 25–6. Suggested Aggressive Protocol After Anterolateral or Anteromedial Extra-Articular Procedures

Postoperative day

1–4
- Hinged postoperative brace (45°)
- Gait: initially non–weight bearing
- Transcutaneous electronic nerve stimulation and ice
- Quadriceps sets
- Hamstrings sets
- Ankle pumps
- Straight leg raises and flexion-to-extension 70° to 40° in the hinged postoperative brace

4–5
- Dressing change
- Immobilizer set 90° to 40°
- Gait: touch-down weight bearing
- Exercises performed in the brace, as above with addition of terminal knee extension, hamstrings curls, hip flexion, and hip extension

10–12
- Stitches out
- Patient allowed to shower
- Immobilizer set 90° to 40°
- Gait: touch-down weight bearing
- Exercises as for days 1 through 5

Postoperative status

3 wk
- Hinged postoperative brace set 90° to 20°
- Gait: partial weight bearing
- Exercises out of brace
- Exercises as for days 1 through 5, plus straight leg raises with terminal knee extensions, flexion to extension 90° to 0°, flexion activities

6 wk
- Hinged postoperative brace set 90° to 10°
- Gait: partial weight bearing to full weight bearing (2 to 4 wk)
- Maintain 10° flexion contracture
- Exercise as at 3 wk
- Biking when range of motion is sufficient
- Well leg and upper body program

12 wk
- Gait: full weight bearing with no brace
- Exercises as at 6 wk
- Side step-ups, swimming program, walking program, weights to 10 pounds as tolerated

4 mo
- Exercises as for 12 wk, plus weight room activities
- More aggressive closed-chain activities

5–7 mo
- Functional activities
- Continued weight bearing
- Weight training
- Progressive running and agility skills
- Return to sport when testing and functional activities are within normal limits

Table 25–7. Rehabilitation After Intra-Articular Patellar Tendon Graft

Immediately postoperative
 Compression dressing, ice
 Locked hinged brace 0° (treat extra-articular or meniscal repair combined with intra-articular reconstruction as intra-articular reconstruction)
 Proper elevation
 Ankle pumps encouraged, muscle stimulation and biofeedback and quadriceps sets
 CPM
Postoperative day 1
 Patient out of bed
 Gait: weight bearing to tolerance
 Ankle pumps
 Quadriceps sets, terminal knee extensions or heel lifts
 Obtain full passive extension out of brace
Postoperative day 2
 Dressing change
 Begin working to 90° of flexion out of brace
 Unlock brace as patient becomes more comfortable
 Gait: weight bearing to tolerance with crutches
 Stimulation to train quadriceps
 Exercises (out of brace): quadriceps sets, heel lifts, flexion activities, straight leg raises with heel lift, hamstrings stretches, passive extension, and full flexion, as tolerated
Postoperative day 3
 Gait: weight bearing to tolerance with crutches
 Exercises out of brace: quadriceps sets, heel lifts, flexion activities, straight leg raises with heel lift, hamstrings stretching, passive extension to 0°, hip flexion, flexion to extension 90° to 45°, active range of motion 90°+ as tolerated, and hamstrings curls
 Functional exercises such as mini-squats and rubber tubing leg presses started and progressed
Status postoperatively 2–3 wks to 6 wks
 Brace 0° to full flexion, decrease use as comfortable, replace with knee sleeve as comfortable
 Gait: weight bearing to tolerance with crutches, progress to full weight bearing as quadriceps develop
 Exercises: biking as tolerated, 30 to 60 minutes
 Gradually increase progressive resistance exercises to 5 pounds on exercises for day 3 above
 90° to 45° flexion to extension for quadriceps training
 Squats as tolerated, step-up standing, knee flexion progressed, hip extension
 Hip abduction, hip adduction
 Rubber tubing, squats (single and double), leg press
 Walking program
 Safe isokinetics
 Proprioception exercises
 Continue exercises from the first 6 wks using weights up to 10 pounds
 Steps

Table 25–7. (*continued*).

Closed-chain activities
Progress proper quadriceps-strengthening activities
Isokinetic testing
Status postoperatively 12 wks
Isokinetic testing
Begin running program as strength and knee conditions permit
Status postoperatively 4–6 mos
Functional brace for support (p.r.n.)
Agility programs
Sport-specific activities
Return to sport when testing and functional activities are within normal limits

Nonsurgically Treated PCL Injuries with PLRI

1. Low stress closed-chain exercises, starting with quadriceps sets, terminal knee extensions, straight leg raises, and exercises for hip flexors, adductors, abductors, and extensors
   a. Avoid hamstrings exercises initially; add once ligament heals
   b. Work quadriceps from 60–0° in flexion-extension mode and in straight leg-raise mode
2. Control weight bearing initially with crutches, progressing as quadriceps control ↑
   a. No brace unless athlete uncomfortable
   b. Progress to functional activities as tolerated
3. For acute injuries, immobilize with extension lock at 20° for up to 6 wks; do above-described exercises without fully extending knee
4. Return to activity when full ROM regained, and strength, power, and endurance equal to uninjured knee

Surgically Treated PCL Injuries with PLRI

1. Direct Repair of PCL
   a. Postop cast (including foot) for 4–6 wks with knee flexed 60–70°
      (1) When elevating leg, support behind tibia (not heel) to avoid PCL-directed force
      (2) Once cast removed, long-leg brace with heel cup takes tibial weight off repair
   b. Bear no weight until quadriceps control regained (8–10 wks postop)
   c. Do quadriceps exercises, but delay hamstrings strengthening until 3 mos after surgery
   d. Start cycling and closed-chain exercises once ROM comfortable and weight-bearing status permits

2. If graft used, protect (especially from posterior shear), but start immediate motion (protocol similar to ACL)
3. Arcuate Complex Advancements
   a. Cast extremity at 60–70° flexion with foot incorporated
      (1) Pelvic band keeps leg from rotating externally and stressing posterolateral corner
      (2) Tibia must be adequately supported and heel must not rest on bed when supine
      (3) Perform quadriceps sets and straight leg raises in cast
   b. At 6 wks, replace cast with long-leg brace with dial-lock hinges and heel cup
      (1) Gain flexion with active-assisted motion
      (2) Gain extension gradually and slowly with active quadriceps contractions
      (3) Initially lock brace at 60°, then lock in further extension as tolerated, but always less than amount of active knee extension to avoid stressing reconstructed structures
   c. Exercises: terminal knee extensions, straight leg raises, limited flexion-extension exercises, and strengthening of hip flexors, adductors, abductors, and extensors; protect knee from shear forces by supporting proximal tibia posteriorly
   d. Start hamstrings strengthening at 12 wks
   e. Allow partial weight bearing once active extension 20°, progressing from toe-heel to heel-toe gait as extension improves
   f. ↑ extension gradually
   g. Once good ROM and stability achieved, use functional continuum
4. As with nonsurgical treatment, return to activity when full ROM regained, and strength, power, and endurance equal to uninjured knee

LOWER LEG INJURIES

Shin Splints

1. Rest (critical for successful resolution of pain), duration depending on symptoms
2. Stretching exercises, careful warm-up, and exercises to regain ROM before athletic activity
3. Correct any biomechanical abnormalities
   a. Easily correct overpronation plus heel valgus with appropriate orthotic
   b. Taping to support longitudinal arch
4. Proper running shoes provide shock absorption and firm heel contour
5. Alternative workouts, superficial hot and cold therapy, and NSAIDs help prepare for important competition

Compartment Syndromes

1. Start ROM exercises of knee, ankle, and foot immediately after surgery
2. Weight bearing as tolerated
3. Regain ROM, strength, endurance, proprioception, power, speed, and agility
4. Rapidly resume normal activities once wound heals

Gastrocnemius-Soleus Complex Injury

1. Immediate partial or nonweight bearing
2. Calf wrap
3. Crutches or cane to bear weight only to point of discomfort, but not to limp: important to maintain pain-free gait
4. With minor injuries, wrap and heel lift to reduce passive dorsiflexion during ambulation often sufficient
5. For more serious injury, continue ISE (ice, stretching, exercise)
   a. Start pool exercises and backward walking early: pressure less during pool walking and dorsiflexion less during backward walking
   b. Follow active dorsiflexion (Fig. 25–20), after gently stretch calf with passive ROM exercises
   c. Use towel to perform resistive plantar flexion exercises
   d. Start standing stretch and flat heel raises, progressing from passive stretching and resistive exercise off step to calf machine (Fig. 25-21)
6. With improvement, remove heel lift and acclimate to flat court or field shoes

ACHILLES TENDINITIS

1. Rehab similar to gastrocnemius-soleus injury
2. 7-day calf-machine regimen
   days 1–2: 3 sets of 10 reps at slow speed with no pain
   days 3–5: moderate speed with no pain
   days 6–7: fast speed with slight discomfort

Achilles Tendon Ruptures

1. Immobilize for 6–8 wks with dorsiflexion block splint or removable protective brace to allow early ROM
2. Sometimes cast protection for 4–6 wks best; start gentle passive and active ROM exercises when cast removed
3. Early, limited, touch-down weight bearing for 3–4 wks, then gradual ↑ to full weight bearing in cast or brace
4. Start progressive resistance exercises as tolerated, continuing ankle flexibility exercises

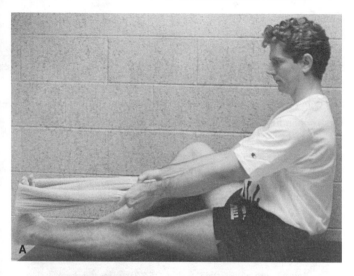

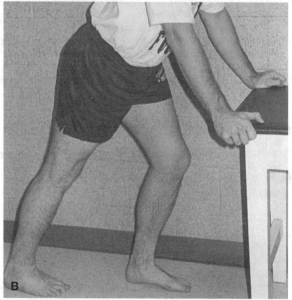

Fig. 25–20. (A, B) Range of motion exercises for dorsiflexion.

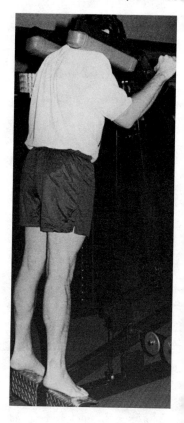

Fig. 25–21. Calf machine exercise for gastrocnemius-soleus strength.

5. To routine gastrocnemius-soleus exercises, add early pool walking (good exercises and well tolerated)
6. Add heavy resistance when ambulation pain free without limping
7. Resume sports activity 4–6 mos after surgery

ANKLE AND FOOT INJURIES

Minor to Moderate Ankle Sprains

1. Start active ROM day after injury and use cryotherapy
   a. Allow only dorsiflexion and plantar flexion: no inversion-eversion
   b. Emphasize heel cord stretching throughout program
2. Progress stretching into dorsiflexion with towel stretches and then wall stretches, first as double leg and then as single leg

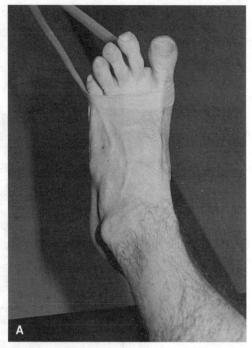

Fig. 25–22. Strengthening exercises for ankle sprains: A. Dorsiflexion strengthening. B. Inversion strengthening. C. Eversion strengthening.

    a. Stretch with knee bent and straight for maximum ROM
    b. Stretch before ankle taped to maintain maximum dorsiflexion
    c. Bicycling and walking down stairs also help regain normal dorsiflexion
3. Strengthening Exercises
    a. Perform isometric exercises in multiple positions (6 sec each) daily; 3 motions (ie, dorsiflexion, inversion, eversion) can be accomplished with elastic tubing (Fig. 25–22)
    b. Add progressive isotonic and isokinetic resistance exercises as tolerated
    c. Manual dynamic resistance also helpful
    d. Plantar flexion requires more extensive exercise to fully regain strength; use heavy weights with few reps (with knee flexed and extended) to restore gastrocnemius-soleus to normal strength
4. Start proprioceptive exercises (eg, tilt board and balance disc) when strength permits

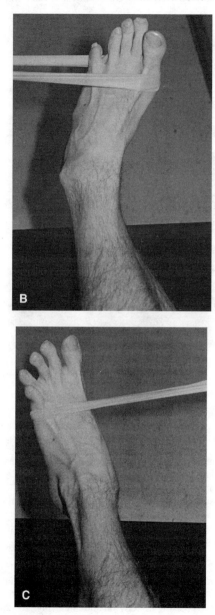

Fig. 25–22. *(continued).*

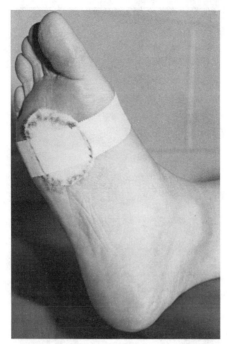

Fig. 25–23. Metatarsal pad.

5. Then perform exercises to ↑ endurance, power, speed, and agility
6. Tape and return to competition when criteria for return to activity met

Longitudinal Arch Strains

1. Towel curls and inversion exercises strengthen toe flexors and posterior tibialis
2. Heel cord stretching important
3. External support provided by taping longitudinal arch; when taping, dorsiflex ankle and flex toes to elevate arch and shorten toe flexors
4. If exercise and taping insufficient, semi-rigid orthotic may be needed, especially with pes planus

Metatarsal Arch Strains

1. Toe flexor exercises and metatarsal pad usually alleviate symptoms
2. Fit pad so metatarsal heads (usually 2 and 3) supported proximally and pad not pressing directly on sore area (Fig. 25–23)
3. May glue pad into shoe or incorporate into orthotic

Plantar Fasciitis

1. Most important: eliminate causative factors by reviewing training techniques and shoe wear
2. Rest, NSAIDs, contrast treatments, and ultrasound provide pain relief
3. Transverse friction massage for 6–8 mins every other day aids healing
4. Heel cord stretching
5. Arch taping may help, especially tight medial pull of tape over posteromedial plantar surface
6. Soft orthotic with deep heel cup (Tuli) and medial heel wedge (and medial arch support for pes planus foot) decreases stress and allows pain-free gait
7. Ankle-foot orthotic night splints with 5° dorsiflexion may help refractory cases

Turf Toe

1. After acute symptoms subside, heat modalities (eg, whirlpool), stretching, active and passive toe motion exercises, and foot-strengthening exercises beneficial
2. Stiff (rigid steel or plastic) orthotic that limits great toe dorsiflexion protects joint

Suggested Readings

Chapter 1

Powell, J.: 636,000 injuries annually in high school football. Athletic Training 22: 19, 1987.

Chapter 2

American Academy of Pediatrics Committee on Sports Medicine: Atlantoaxial instability in Down syndrome. Pediatrics 74: 152, 1984.

American Academy of Pediatrics Committee on Sports Medicine: Recommendations for participation in competitive sports. Pediatrics, 81: 737, 1988.

Bergfeld, J., et al.: Preparticipation Physical Evaluation Monograph. Kansas City, American Academy of Family Physicians, 1992.

Eichner, E.R.: Infection, immunity, and exercise. Physician Sportsmed. 21(1): 125, 1993.

Feinstein, R.A., Soileau, E.J., and Daniel, W.A. Jr.: A national survey of preparticipation physical examination requirements. Physician Sportsmed. 16(5): 51, 1988.

Foster, C.: Physiologic testing: Does it help the athlete? Physician Sportsmed. 17(10): 103, 1989.

Kibler, W.B., Chandler, T.J., Uhl, T., and Maddux, R.F.: A musculoskeletal approach to the preparticipation physical examination. Preventing injury and improving performance. Am J. Sports Med. 17: 525, 1989.

Lombardo, J.A.: Preparticipation evaluation. In The Pediatric Athlete. Edited by J.A. Sullivan and W.A. Grana. Park Ridge, IL, American Academy of Orthopaedic Surgeons, 1988.

Magnes, S.A., Henderson, J.M., and Hunter, S.C.: What conditions limit sports participation?: Experience with 10,540 athletes. Physician Sportsmed. 20(5): 113, 1992.

Mitchell, J.H., Maron, B.J., and Epstein, S.E.: 16th Bethesda Conference: Cardiovascular abnormalities in the athlete: Recommendations regarding eligibility for competition. J. Am Coll. Cardiol. 6: 1186, 1985.

Chapter 3

Auerbach, P.S., and Geehr, E.C. (eds.): Management of Wilderness and Environmental Emergencies. 2nd Ed. St. Louis, C.V. Mosby, 1989.

Bracker, M.D.: Environmental and thermal injury. Clin. Sports Med. 11: 419, 1992.

Delaney, K.A.: Heatstroke: Underlying processes and lifesaving management. Postgrad. Med. 91: 379, 1992.

High altitude sickness. Med Lett. 30: 89, 1988.

Levine, B.D.: By what physiological mechanism is dexamethasone beneficial in the prevention of acute mountain sickness. West. J. Med. 4: 106, 1993.

Millard-Stafford, M.: Fluid replacement during exercise in the heat; review and recommendations. Sports Med. 13: 223, 1992.

Robinson, W.: Competing with the cold. Part II. Hypothermia. Physician Sportsmed. 20(1): 61, 1992.

Robinson, W.: Competing with the cold: Part I. Frostbite. Physician Sportsmed. 19(12) 19, 1991.

Squire, D.L.: Heat illness: Fluid and electrolyte issues for pediatric and adolescent athletes. Pediatr. Clin. North Am. 37: 5, 1990.

Tso, F.: High altitude illness. Emerg. Med. Clin. North Am. 10: 231, 1992.

Chapter 4

Bakland, L.K., and Boyne, P.J.: Trauma to the oral cavity. Clin. Sports Med. 8: 25, 1989.

Cantu, R.C.: When to return to contact sports after a cerebral concussion. Sports Med. Digest. 10: 1, 1988.

Dempsey, R.J., and Schneider, R.C.: The management of head injuries in sports. In: Sports Injuries: Mechanisms, Prevention, and Treatment. Edited by R.C. Schneider, et al. Baltimore, Williams & Wilkins, 1985.

Dimeff, R.J., and Hough, D.O.: Preventing cauliflower ear with a modified tie-through technique. Physician Sportsmed. 17(3): 167, 1989.

Erie, J.C.: Eye injuries. Prevention, evaluation, and treatment. Physician Sportsmed. 19(11): 108, 1991.

Kelly, J.P., et al.: Concussion in sports: Guidelines for the prevention of catastrophic outcome. J.A.M.A. 266: 2867, 1991.

Schendel, S.A.: Sports-related nasal injuries. Physician Sportsmed. 18(10): 59, 1990.

Schultz, R.C., and de Camara, D.L.: Athletic facial injuries. J.A.M.A. 252: 3395, 1984.

Shell, D., Carico, G.A., and Patton, R.M.: Can subdural hematoma result from repeated minor head injury? Physician Sportsmed. 21(4): 74, 1993.

Wilberger, J.E., Jr., and Maroon, J.C.: Head injuries in athletes. Clin. Sports Med. 8: 1, 1989.

Chapter 5

Bergqvist, D., Hedelin, H., Lindblad, B., and Mätzsch, T.: Abdominal injuries in children: an analysis of 348 cases. Injury 16: 217, 1985.

Diamond, D.L.: Sports-related abdominal trauma. J. Trauma 8: 91, 1989.

Espinosa, R., Badui, E., Castaño, R., and Madrid, R.: Acute posteroinferior wall myocardial infarction secondary to football chest trauma. Chest 88: 928, 1985.

Groskin, S.: The radiologic evaluation of chest pain in the athlete. Clin. Sports Med. 6: 845, 1987.

Kenney, P.: Abdominal pain in athletes. Clin. Sports Med. 6: 885, 1986.

Lehman, R.C.: Thoracoabdominal musculoskeletal injuries in racquet sports. Clin. Sports Med. 7: 267, 1988.

McEntire, J.E., Hess, W.E., and Coleman, S.S.: Rupture of the pectoralis major muscle. J. Bone Joint Surg. *54A:* 1040, 1972.

Mellion, M.B., Walsh, W.M., and Shelton, G.L.: The Team Physician's Handbook. Philadelphia, Hanley & Belfus, 1990.

Rose, K.D., Stone, F., Fuenning, S.J., and Williams, J.: Cardiac contusion resulting from "spearing" in football. Arch. Internal Med. 118: 129, 1966.

Scharplatz, D., Thurleman, K., and Enderlin, F.: Thoracoabdominal trauma in ski accidents. Injury *10:* 86, 1978.

Chapter 6

Bergfeld, W.F.: Dermatologic problems in athletes. Clin. Sports Med. 1: 419, 1982.

Conklin, R.J.: Common cutaneous disorders in athletes. Sports Med. 9: 100, 1990.

Garal, T., Hrisonalost, and Rink, L.: Transmission of infectious agents during athletic competition, a report to all national government bodies by the U.S. Olympic Committee Sports Medicine and Science Committee. Colorado Springs, U.S. Olympic Committee, 1991.

Kantor, G.R., and Bergfeld, W.F.: Common and uncommon dermatologic diseases related to sports activities. Dermatol. Dis. Sport 1: 225, 1990.

Kaplan, E.L. and Hill, H.R.: Return of rheumatic fever. Consequences, implications, and needs. J. Pediatr. 111: 244, 1987.

Laperiere, A., Antoni, M.H., and Fletcher, M.A.: Exercise and health maintenance in AIDS. In Clinical Assessment and Treatment in HIV. Rehabilitation of a Chronic Illness. Edited by M.L. Galantino. Thorofare, NJ, Charles B. Slack, 1992.

Ramsey, M.L.: Athlete's foot: Clinical update. Physician Sportsmed. 17 (10): 78, 1989.

Shepherd, R.J., et al.: Physical activity and the immune system. Can. J. Sports Sci. 16: 163, 1991.

Steere, A.C.: Current understanding of Lyme disease. Hosp. Pract. 28 (4): 37, 1993.

Treatment of sexually transmitted diseases. Med. Lett. 32: 5, 1990.

Chapter 7

AAP issues statement on exercise induced asthma in children. Am Fam. Physician. 40: 314, 1989.

Afrasiabi, R., and Spector, S.L.: Exercise-induced asthma. Physician Sportsmed.19 (5): 49, 1991.

Blackett, P.R.: Child and adolescent athletes with diabetes. Physician Sportsmed. 16 (3): 133, 1988.

Drugs for ambulatory asthma. Med. Lett. 35: 11, 1993.

LaPorte, R.E., Dorman, J.S., Tajima, N., et al.: Pittsburgh Insulin-Dependent Diabetes Mellitus Morbidity and Mortality Study: Physical activity and diabetic complications. Pediatrics 78: 1027, 1986.

McCarthy, P.: Wheezing or breezing through exercise-induced asthma. Physician Sportsmed. 17 (7): 125, 1989.

McFadden, E.: Fatal and near-fatal asthma. N. Engl. J. Med. 324: 409, 1991.

National Institutes of Health Consensus Development Conference on Diet and Exercise in Non-Insulin Dependent Diabetes Mellitus, draft statement. Bethesda, MD, National Institute of Diabetes and Digestive and Kidney Diseases and the National Institutes of Health Office of Medical Application of Research, 1986.

Robbins, D.C., and Carleton, S.: Managing the diabetic athlete. Physician Sportsmed. 17 (12): 45, 1989.

The Diabetes Control and Complications Trial Research Group: The effect of intensive treatment of diabetes on the development and progression of long-term complications in insulin-dependent diabetes mellitus. N. Engl. J. Med. 329: 977, 1993.

Chapter 8

Buori, I., Makarainem, M., and Jaaskelainem, A.: Sudden death and physical activity. Cardiology 63: 287, 1987.

Cantu, R. C.: Congenital cardiovascular disease—the major cause for athletic death in high school and college. Med. Sci. Sports Exerc. 24: 279, 1992.

Davies, M. J.: Anatomic features in victims of sudden coronary death. Circulation 85 (Suppl. I): 1–19, 1992.

Frenneaux, M. P., et al.: Determinants of exercise capacity in hypertrophic cardiomyopathy. J. Am. Coll. Cardiol. 13: 1521, 1989.

Jeresaty, R. M.: Mitral valve prolapse: Implications for the athlete. In Cardiovascular Evaluation of Athletes. Edited by B. F. Waller and W. P. Harvey. Newton, NJ, Laennec, 1992.

Klitzner, T. S.: Sudden cardiac death in children. Circulation 82: 629, 1990.

Maron, B. J., et al.: Results of screening a large group of intercollegiate competitive athletes for cardiovascular disease. J. Am Coll. Cardiol. 10: 1214, 1987.

Mitchell, J. H., Maron, B. J., and Epstein, S. E.: 16th Bethesda Conference: Cardiovascular abnormalities in the athlete: Recommendations regarding eligibility for competition. J. Am. Coll. Cardiol. 6: 1186, 1985.

Neuspiel, D. R., and Kuller, L. H.: Sudden and unexpected natural death in childhood and adolescence. J. A. M. A. 254: 1321, 1985.

Phillips, M., et al.: Sudden cardiac death in air force recruits. J. A. M. A. 256: 2696, 1986.

Chapter 9

Boxall, D., Bradford, D.S., Winter, R.B., and Moe, J.H.: Management of severe spondylolisthesis in children and adolescents. J. Bone Joint Surg. 61A: 479, 1979.

Burkus, J.K., and Denis, F.: Thoracic disc disease. In Chapman, M.W.(ed.): Operative Orthopaedics, 2nd Ed. Philadelphia, J.B. Lippincott, 1993.

Hershman, E.B.: Brachial plexus injuries. Clin. Sports Med. 9: 311, 1990.

Lowe, T.G.: Scheuermann disease. J. Bone Joint Surg. 72A: 940, 1990.

Micheli, L.J.: Low back pain in the adolescent: differential diagnosis. Am. J. Sports Med. 7: 362, 1979.

Speer, K.P., Bassett, F.H.: The prolonged burner syndrome. Am. J. Sports Med. 18: 591, 1990.

Torg, J.S. et al.: The National Football Head and Neck Injury Registry. Report and conclusion 1978. J.A.M.A. 241: 1477, 1979.

Torg, J.S., and Das, M.: Trampoline-related quadriplegia: Review of the literature and reflections on the American Academy of Pediatrics position statement. Pediatrics 74: 804, 1984.

Torg, J.S.: Epidemiology, pathomechanics, and prevention of athletic injuries to the cervical spine. Med. Sci. Sports Exerc. 17: 295, 1985.

Vereschagin, K.S., Wiens, J.J., Fanton, G.S., and Dillingham, M.F.: Burners, don't overlook or underestimate them. Physician Sportsmed. 19(9): 96, 1991.

Chapter 10

Curtis, R.J. Jr.: Operative management of children's fractures of the shoulder region. Orthop. Clin. North Am. 21: 315, 1990.

Hagg, O., and Lundberg, B.: Aspects of prognostic factors in comminuted and dislocated proximal humeral fractures. In Surgery of the Shoulder. Edited by J.E. Bateman, and R.P. Welsh. Philadelphia, B.C. Decker, 1984.

Larsen, E., Bjerg-Nielsen, A., and Christensen, P.: Conservative or surgical treatment of acromioclavicular dislocation. J. Bone Joint Surg. 68A: 552, 1986.

Richards, R.R.: Acromioclavicular joint injuries. AAOS Instr. Course Lect. 42: 259, 1993.

Rockwood, C.A. Jr., and Matsen, F.A. III (eds.): The Shoulder. Philadelphia, W.B. Saunders, 1990.

Rockwood, C.A. Jr., Wilkins, K.E., and King, R.E. (eds.): Fractures in Children. 3rd Ed. Philadelphia, J.B. Lippincott, 1991.

Silloway, K.A., et al.: Clavicular fractures and acromioclavicular joint injuries in lacrosse: Preventable injuries. J. Emerg. Med. 3: 117, 1985.

Thompson, D.A., Flynn, T.C., Miller, P.W., and Fischer, R.P.: The significance of scapular fractures. J. Trauma 25: 974, 1985.

Warren, R.F.: The acromioclavicular and sternoclavicular joints. In Surgery of the Musculoskeletal System. 2nd Ed. Edited by C.M. Evarts. New York, Churchill Livingstone, 1990.

Wojtys, E.M., and Nelson, G.: Conservative treatment of grade III acromioclavicular dislocations. Clin. Orthop. 268: 112, 1991.

Chapter 11

Andrews, J.R., Carson, W.G. Jr., and McLeod, W.D.: Glenoid labrum tears related to the long head of the biceps. Am. J. Sports Med. 13: 337, 1985.

Caspari, R.B., and Geissler, W.B.: Arthroscopic manifestations of shoulder subluxation and dislocation. Clin. Orthop. 291: 54, 1993.

Esch, J.C. Surgical arthroscopy of the shoulder: Anterior instability. In Arthroscopic Surgery. The Shoulder and Elbow. Edited by J.C. Esch and C.L. Baker. Philadelphia, J.B. Lippincott, 1993.

Jobe, F.W., and Kvitne, R.S.: Shoulder pain in the overhand or throwing athlete. Orthop. Rev. 18: 963, 1989.

Matsen, F.A. III(ed.): The Shoulder. A Balance of Mobility and Stability. Rosemont, IL, American Academy of Orthopaedic Surgeons, 1993.

Mellion, M.B., Walsh, W.M., and Shelton, G.L.: The Team Physician's Handbook. Philadelphia, Hanley & Belfus, 1990.

Pappas, A.M., Goss, T.P., and Kleinman, P.K.: Symptomatic shoulder instability due to lesions of the glenoid labrum. Am.J. Sports Med. 11: 279, 1983.

Rockwood, C.A. Jr., and Matsen, F.A. III (eds.): The Shoulder. Philadelphia, W.B. Saunders, 1990.

Snyder, S.J., et al.: SLAP lesions of the shoulder. Arthroscopy 6: 274, 1990.

Turkel, S.J., Panio, M.W., Marshall, J.L., and Girgis, F.G.: Stabilizing mechanisms preventing anterior dislocation of the glenohumeral joint. J. Bone Joint Surg. 63A: 120, 1981.

Chapter 12

Apoil, A., and Augerean, B.: Anterosuperior arthrolysis of the shoulder for rotatory cuff degenerative lesions. In Surgery of the Shoulder. Edited by M. Post, B.F. Morrey, and R.J. Hawkins. St. Louis, Mosby-Year Book, 1990.

Bigliani, L.U., Morrison, D., and April, E.W.: The morphology of the acromion and its relationship to rotator cuff tears. Orthop. Trans. 10: 228, 1986.

Fukuda, H., et al.: The partial thickness tear of the rotator cuff. Orthop. Trans. 7:137, 1983.

Hawkins, R.J., Misamore, G.W., and Hobeika, P.E.: Surgery for full-thickness rotator-cuff tears. J. Bone Joint Surg. 67A:1349, 1985.

Matsen, F.A. III, and Arntz, C.T.: Rotator cuff tendon failure. In The Shoulder. Edited by C.A. Rockwood Jr., and F.A. Matsen III. Philadelphia, W.B. Saunders, 1990.

Neer, C.S. II: Anterior acromioplasty for the chronic impingement syndrome in the shoulder. A preliminary report. J. Bone Joint Surg. 54A: 41, 1972.

Neer, C.S. II: Impingement lesions. Clin. Orthop. 173: 30, 1983.

Rockwood, C.A., and Lyons, F.R.: Shoulder impingement syndrome. Diagnosis, radiographic evaluation, and treatment with a modified Neer acromioplasty. J. Bone Joint Surg. 75A: 409, 1993.

Watson, M.: Major ruptures of the rotator cuff: The results of surgical repair in 89 patients. J. Bone Joint Surg. 67B: 618, 1985.

Yamanaka, K., Fukuda, H., Hamada, K., and Mikasa, M.: Incomplete thickness tears of the rotation cuff. Orthop. Traumatol. Surg. 26: 713, 1983.

Chapter 13

Bernstein, S.M., King, J.D., and Sanderson, R.A.: Fractures of the medial epicon-dyle of the humerus. Contemp. Orthop. 3: 637, 1981.

Mehlhoff, T.I., Noble, P.C., Bennett, J.B., and Tullos, H.S.: Simple dislocation of the elbow in the adult. J. Bone Joint Surg. 70A: 244, 1988.

Morrey, B.F., An, K.N., and Stormont, T.J.: Force transmission through the radial head. J. Bone Joint Surg. 70A: 250, 1988.

Morrey, B.F., and An, K.N.: Articular and ligamentous contributions to the stabil-ity of the elbow joint. Am. J. Sports Med. 11: 315, 1983.

Morrey, B.F., and An, K.N.: Functional anatomy of the ligaments of the elbow. Clin. Orthop. 201: 84, 1985.

Morrey, B.F., Tanaka, S., and An, K.N.: Valgus stability of the elbow. Clin. Orthop. 265: 187, 1991.

O'Driscoll, S.W., Bell, D.F., and Morrey, B.F.: Posterolateral rotatory instability of the elbow. J. Bone Joint Surg. 73A: 440, 1991.

Schwab, G.H., Bennett, J.B., Woods, G.W., and Tullos, H.S.: Biomechanics of elbow instability. The role of the medial collateral ligament. Clin. Orthop. 146: 42, 1980.

Wilson, N.I.L., Ingram, R., Rymaszewski, L., and Miller, J.H.: Treatment of fractures of the medial epicondyle of the humerus. Injury 19: 342, 1988.

Woods, G.W., and Tullos, H.S.: Elbow instability and medial epicondyle frac-tures. Am. J. Sports Med. 5: 23, 1977.

Chapter 14

Andrews, J.R., and Wilson, F.: Valgus extension overload in the pitching elbow. In Injuries to the Throwing Arm. Edited by B. Zarins, J.R. Andrews, and W.G. Carson Jr. Philadelphia, W.B. Saunders, 1985.

Berkeley, M.E., Bennett, J.B., and Woods, G.W.: Surgical management of acute and chronic elbow problems. In Injuries to the Throwing Arm. Edited by B. Zarins, J.R. Andrews, and W.G. Carson Jr. Philadelphia, W.B. Saunders, 1985.

Cabrera, J.M., and McCue, F.C. III: Nonosseous athletic injuries of the elbow, forearm, and hand. Clin. Sports Med. 5: 681, 1986.

Carson, W.G. Jr.: Arthroscopy of the elbow. Instr. Course Lect. 37:195, 1988.

Jobe, F.W., and Nuber, G.: Throwing injuries of the elbow. Clin. Sports Med. 5: 621, 1986.

Morrey, B.F., An, K.N., and Chao, E.Y.S.: Functional evaluation of the elbow.

In The Elbow and Its Disorders. Edited by B.F. Morrey. Philadelphia, W.B. Saunders, 1985.

Nirschl, R.P.: Elbow tendinosis/tennis elbow. Clin. Sports Med. 11: 851, 1992.

Posner, M.A.: Compressive neuropathies of the median and radial nerves at the elbow. Clin. Sports Med. 9: 343, 1990.

Singer, K.M., and Roy, S.P.: Osteochondrosis of the humeral capitellum. Am. J. Sports Med. 12: 351, 1984.

Wilson, F.D., Andrews, J.R., Blackburn, T.A., and McCluskey, G.: Valgus extension overload in the pitching elbow. Am. J. Sports Med. 11: 83, 1983.

Chapter 15

Kahler, D.M., and McCue, F.C. III: Metacarpophalangeal and proximal interphalangeal joint injuries of the hand, including the thumb. Clin. Sports Med. 11: 57, 1992.

Linscheid, R.L., and Dobyns, J.H.: Athletic injuries of the wrist. Clin. Orthop. 198: 141, 1985.

McCue, F.C., et al.: The coach's finger. J. Sports Med. 2: 270, 1974.

McCue, F.C., et al.: Ulnar collateral ligament injuries of the thumb in athletes. J. Sports Med. 2: 70, 1974.

Rodriguez, A.L.: Injuries to the collateral ligaments of the proximal interphalangeal joints. Hand 5: 66, 1990.

Taleisnik, J.: The ligaments of the wrist. J. Hand Surg. 1: 110, 1976.

Taleisnik, J.: Wrist: Anatomy, function and injury. Course Lect. 27: 61, 1978.

Terzis, J.K., and Smith, K.L.: The Peripheral Nerve: Structure, Function, and Reconstruction. New York, Raven Press, 1990.

Whipple, T.L.: The role of arthroscopy in the treatment of wrist injuries in the athlete. Clin. Sports Med. 11: 227, 1992.

Zemel, N.P., and Stark, H.H.: Fractures and dislocations of the carpal bones. Clin. Sports Med. 5: 709, 1986.

Chapter 16

Cooper, D.E., Warren, R.F., and Barnes, R.: Traumatic subluxation of the hip resulting in aseptic necrosis and chondrolysis in a professional football player. Am. J. Sports Med. 19: 322, 1991.

Frost, A., and Bauer, M.: Skier's hip—a new clinical entity? J. Orthop. Trauma 5: 47, 1991.

Fullerton, L.R. Jr., and Snowdy, H.A.: Femoral neck stress fractures. Am. J. Sports Med. 16: 365, 1988.

Mandell, G.A., Keret, D., Harcke, T., and Bowen, J.R.: Chondrolysis: detection by bone scintigraphy. J. Pediatr. Orthop. 12: 80, 1992.

Offierski, C.M.: Traumatic dislocation of the hip in children. J. Bone Joint Surg. 63B: 194, 1981.

Pavlov, H., Nelson, T.L., and Warren, R.F.: Stress fractures of the pubic ramus. A report of twelve cases. J. Bone Joint Surg. 64A: 1020, 1982.

Pavlov, H.: Roentgen examination of groin and hip pain in the athlete. Clin. Sports Med. 6: 829, 1987.

Renstrom, P., and Peterson, L.: Groin injuries in athletes. Br. J. Sports Med. 14: 30, 1980.

Rosenthal, R.E., and Coker, W.L.: Posterior fracture-dislocation of the hip: An epidemiologic review. J. Trauma 19: 572, 1979.

Waters, P.M., and Millis, M.B.: Hip and pelvic injuries in the young athlete. Clin. Sports Med. 7: 513, 1988.

Chapter 17

Cook, S.D., Kester, M.A., Brunet, M.E., and Haddal, R.J. Jr.: Biomechanics of running shoe performance. Clin. Sports Med. 4: 619, 1985.

Cox, J.S.: Patellofemoral problems in runners. Clin. Sports Med. 4: 699, 1985.

Curwin, S., and Stanish, W.D.: Tendinitis: Its Etiology and Treatment. Lexington, MA, Collamore Press, 1984.

Ferretti, A., Puddu, G., Mariani, P.P., and Neri, M.: Jumper's knee: An epidemiological study of volleyball players. Physician Sportsmed. 12 (10): 97, 1984.

Garrett, W.E. Jr., et al.: The effect of muscle architecture on the biomechanical failure properties of skeletal muscle under passive extension. Am. J. Sports Med. 16: 7, 1988.

Haas, S.B., and Callaway, H.: Disruptions of the extensor mechanism. Orthop. Clin. North Am. 23: 687, 1992.

Ishikawa, K., Kai, K., and Mizuta, H.: Avulsion of the hamstring muscles from the ischial tuberosity: A report of two cases. Clin. Orthop. 232: 153, 1988.

Martinez, S.F., Steingard, M.A., and Steingard, P.M.: Thigh compartment syndrome—a limb-threatening emergency. Physician Sportsmed. 21 (3): 94, 1993.

Rupani, H.D., Holder, L.E., Espinola, D.A., and Engin, S.L.: Three-phase radionuclide bone imaging in sports medicine. Radiology 156: 187, 1985.

Sommer, H.M.: Patellar chondropathy and apicitis, and muscle imbalances of the lower extremities in competitive sports. Sports Med. 5: 386:1988.

Chapter 18

Hughston, J.C., and Walsh, W.M.: Proximal and distal reconstruction of the extensor mechanism for patellar subluxation. Clin. Orthop. 144: 36, 1979.

Hughston, J.C., Walsh, W.M., and Puddu, G.: Patellar Subluxation and Dislocation. Philadelphia, W.B. Saunders, 1984.

Hughston, J.C.: Subluxation of the patella. J. Bone Joint Surg. 50A: 1003, 1968.

Kolowich, P.A., Paulos, L.E., Rosenberg, T.D., and Farnsworth, S.: Lateral release of the patella: Indications and contraindications. Am. J. Sports Med. 18: 359, 1990.

McConnell, J.: The management of chondromalacia patellae: A long term solution. Austr. J. Physiother. 2: 215, 1986.

Minkoff, J., and Fein, L.: The role of radiography in the evaluation and treatment of common anarthrotic disorders of the patellofemoral joint. Clin. Sports Med. 8: 203, 1989.

Shelton, G.L., and Thigpen, L.K.: Rehabilitation of patellofemoral dysfunction: A review of the literature. J. Orthop. Sports Phys. Ther. 14: 243, 1991.

Turba, J.E., Walsh, W.M., and McLeod, W.D.: Long-term results of extensor mechanism reconstruction. A standard for evaluation. Am. J. Sports Med. 7: 91, 1979.

Vainionpaa, S., et al.: Acute dislocation of the patella. A prospective review of operative treatment. J. Bone Joint Surg. 72B: 366, 1990.

Walsh, W.M.: The patellofemoral joint. In Orthopaedic Sports Medicine: Principles and Practice. Edited by J.C. DeLee and D. Drez. Philadelphia, W.B. Saunders, 1994.

Chapter 19

Arnoczky, S., et al.: Meniscus. In Injury and Repair of the Musculoskeletal Soft Tissues. Edited by S.L. Woo and J.A. Buckwalter. Park Ridge, IL, American Academy of Orthopaedic Surgeons, 1988.

Dandy, D.J.: Chondral and osteochondral lesions of the femoral condyles. In

Knee Surgery: Current Practice. Edited by P.M. Aichroth and W.D. Cannon. New York, Raven Press, 1992.

DeHaven, K, E., Black, K.P., and Griffiths, H.J.: Open meniscus repair technique and two to nine year results. Am. J. Sports Med. 17: 788, 1989.

Hughston, J.C., Hergenroder, P.T., and Courtenay, B.G.: Osteochondritis dissecans of the femoral condyles. J. Bone Joint Surg. 66A: 1340, 1984.

Mankin, H.J.: The reaction of articular cartilage to injury and osteoarthritis. Part I. N. Engl. J. Med. 291: 1285, 1974.

Mankin, H.J.: The reaction of articular cartilage to injury and osteoarthritis. Part II. N. Engl. J. Med. 291: 1335, 1974.

Poehling, G.G., Ruch, D.S., and Chabon, S.J: The landscape of meniscal injuries. Clin. Sports Med. 9: 539, 1990.

Renstrom, P., and Johnson, R.J.: Anatomy and biomechanics of the menisci. Clin. Sports Med. 9: 523, 1990.

Selesnick, F.H., et al.: Internal derangement of the knee: Diagnosis by arthrography, arthroscopy, and arthrotomy. Clin. Orthop. 198: 26, 1985.

Terry, G.C., Flandry, F., VanManen, J.W., and Norwood, L.A.: Isolated chondral fractures of the knee. Clin. Orthop. 234: 170, 1988.

Chapter 20

Barrett, G.R., and Savoie, F. II: Operative management of acute PCL injuries with associated pathology: Long-term results. Orthopedics 14: 687, 1991.

Clancy, W.G. Jr., Ray, J.M., and Zoltan, D.J.: Acute tears of the anterior cruciate ligament: Surgical versus conservative treatment. J. Bone Joint Surg. 70A: 1483, 1988.

Cross, M.J., and Powell, J.F.: Longterm followup of a posterior cruciate ligament rupture: A study of 116 cases. Am. J. Sports Med. 12: 292, 1984.

Hughston, J.C., Andrews, J.R., Cross, M.J., and Moschi, A.: Classification of knee ligamentous instabilities. Part I. The medial compartment and cruciate ligaments. J. Bone Joint Surg. 58A: 159, 1976.

Hughston, J.C., Andrews, J.R., Cross, M.J., and Moschi, A.: Classification of knee ligament instabilities. Part II. The lateral compartment. J. Bone Joint Surg. 58A: 173, 1976.

Jackson, R.W.: The torn ACL: Natural history of untreated lesions and rationale for selective treatment. In The Crucial Ligaments. Edited by J.A. Feagin Jr. New York, Churchill Livingstone, 1988.

Johnson, R.J., Beynnon, B.D., Nichols, C.E., and Renstrom, P.A.: Current concepts review—the treatment of injuries of the anterior cruciate ligament. J. Bone Joint Surg. 74A: 140, 1992.

Kurosaka, M., Yoshiya, S., and Andrish, J.T.: A biomechanical comparison of different surgical techniques of graft fixation in anterior cruciate ligament reconstruction. Am. J. Sports Med. 15: 225, 1987.

Noyes, F.R., Matthews, D.S., Mooar, P.A., and Grood, E.S.: The symptomatic anterior cruciate-deficient knee. Part II: The results of rehabilitation, activity modification, and counseling on functional disability. J. Bone Joint Surg. 65A: 163, 1983.

Noyes, F.R., Mooar, P.A., Matthews, D.S., and Butler, D.L.: The symptomatic anterior cruciate-deficient knee. Part I: The long-term functional disability in athletically active individuals. J. Bone Joint Surg. 65A: 154, 1983.

Chapter 21

Baker, C.L., Norwood, L.A., and Hughston, J.C.: Acute posterolateral rotatory instability of the knee. J. Bone Joint Surg. 65A: 614, 1983.

Clancy, W.G. Jr.: Repair and reconstruction of the posterior cruciate ligament. In Operative Orthopaedics. 2nd Ed. Edited by M.W. Chapman. Philadelphia, J.B. Lippincott, 1993.

Gollehon, D.L., Torzilli, P.A., and Warren, R.F.: The role of the posterolateral and cruciate ligaments in the stability of the human knee. J. Bone Joint Surg. 69A: 233, 1987.

Hughston, J.C., Andrews, J.R., Cross, M.J., and Moschi, A.: Classification of knee ligament instabilities. Parts I and II. J. Bone Joint Surg. 58A: 159, 1976.

Hughston, J.C.: Knee Ligaments: Injury and Repair. St. Louis, Mosby-Year Book, 1993.

Indelicato, P.A., Hermansdorfer, J., and Huegel, M.: Nonoperative management of complete tears of the medial collateral ligament of the knee in intercollegiate football players. Clin. Orthop. 256: 174, 1990.

Müller, W.: The Knee: Form, Function and Ligament Reconstruction. New York, Springer-Verlag, 1983.

Seebacher, J.R., et al.: The structure and function of the posterolateral aspect of the knee. J. Bone Joint Surg. 64A: 536, 1982.

Woo, S.L.Y., et al.: The biomechanical and morphological changes in the medial collateral ligament of the rabbit after immobilization and remobilization. J. Bone Joint Surg. 69A: 1200, 1987.

Chapter 22

Bleichrodt, R.P., Kingma, L.M., Binnendijk, B., and Klein, J.P.: Injuries of the lateral ankle ligaments: Classification with tenography and arthrography. Radiology 173: 347, 1989.

Cass, J.R., and Morrey, B.F.: Ankle instability: Current concepts, diagnosis, and treatment. Mayo Clin. Proc. 59: 165, 1984.

Clanton, T.O., Butler, J.E., and Eggert, A.: Injuries to the metatarsophalangeal joints in athletes. Foot Ankle 7: 162, 1986.

DeLee, J.C.: Fractures and dislocations of the foot. In Surgery of the Foot and Ankle. 6th Ed. Edited by R.A. Mann and M.J. Coughlin. St. Louis, C.V. Mosby, 1993.

Hopkinson, W.J., et al.: Syndesmosis sprains of the ankle. Foot Ankle 10: 325, 1990.

Kannus, P., and Renstrom, P.: Treatment for acute tears of the lateral ligaments of the ankle joint. J. Bone Joint Surg. 73A: 305, 1991.

Mann, R.A.: Biomechanics of the foot and ankle. In Surgery of the Foot and Ankle. 6th Ed. Edited by R.A. Mann and M.J. Coughlin. St. Louis, C.V. Mosby, 1993.

Rijke, A.M., Jones, B., and Vierhout, P.A.M.: Stress examination of traumatized lateral ligaments of the ankle. Clin. Orthop. 210: 143, 1986.

Rockwood, C.A., Green, D.P., and Bucholz, R.W.: Fractures in Adults. 3rd Ed. Philadelphia, J.B. Lippincott, 1991.

Storemont, D.M., Morrey, B.F., An, K.N., and Cass, J.R.: Stability of the loaded ankle: Relation between articular restraint and primary and secondary static restraints. Am. J. Sports Med. 13: 295, 1985.

Chapter 23

Alexander, I.J., Johnson, K.A., and Parr, J.W.: Morton's neuroma: A review of recent concepts. Orthopedics 10: 103, 1987.

Bordelon, R.L.: Management of disorders of the forefoot and toenails associated with running. Clin. Sports Med. 4: 717, 1985.

Carter, T.R., Fowler, P.J., and Blockker, C.: Functional postoperative treatment of Achilles tendon repair. Am. J. Sports Med. 20: 459, 1992.

Crosby, L., and McMullen, S.: Heel pain in an active adolescent? Consider calcaneal apophysitis. Physician Sportsmed. 21(4): 89, 1993.

Galloway, M.T., Jokl, P., and Dayton, O.W.: Achilles tendon overuse injuries. Clin. Sports Med. 11: 771, 1992.

Jackson, D.L., and Haglund, B.: Tarsal tunnel syndrome in athletes. Am. J. Sports Med. 19: 61, 1991.

Mannarino, F., and Sexson, S.: The significance of intracompartmental pressures in the diagnosis of chronic exertional compartment syndrome. Orthopedics 12: 1415, 1989.

Rorabeck, C.H., Fowler, P.J., and Nott, L.: The results of fasciotomy in the management of chronic exertional compartment syndrome. Am. J. Sports Med. 16: 224, 1988.

Sammarco, G.J.: Turf toe. Instr. Course Lect. 42: 207, 1993.

Schepsis, A., Leach, R.E., and Gorzyca, J.: Plantar fasciitis. Etiology, treatment, surgical results, and review of the literature. Clin. Orthop. 266: 185, 1991.

Chapter 24

Beck, C., Drez, D. Jr., et al.: Instrumented testing of functional knee braces. Am. J. Sports Med. 14: 253, 1986.

Drez, D.J. Jr. (Ed.): American Academy of Orthopaedic Surgeons: Knee Braces-Seminar Report. Chicago, IL, American Academy of Orthopaedic Surgeons, 1984.

Erie, J.C.: Eye injuries-prevention, evaluation, and treatment. Physician Sportsmed. 19(11) 108, 1991.

France, E.P., et al.: The biomechanics of lateral knee bracing. Part II. Impact response of the braced knee. Am. J. Sports Med. 15: 430, 1987.

Grace, T.G., et al.: Prophylactic knee braces and injury to the lower extremity. J. Bone Joint Surg. 70A: 422, 1988.

Houston, M.E., and Goemans, P.H.: Leg muscle performance of athletes with and without knee support braces. Arch. Phys. Med. Rehabil. 63: 431, 1982.

Mellion, M.B., Walsh, W.M., and Shelton, G.L.: The Team Physician's Handbook. Philadelphia, Hanley & Belfus, 1990.

Paulos, L.E., et al.: Biomechanics of lateral knee bracing. Part I. Response of the valgus restraints to loading. Am. J. Sports Med. 15: 419, 1987.

Smith, C.R.: Mouth guards take a bite out of injuries. Physician Sportsmed. 20(7): 23, 1992.

Steele, B.E.: Protective pads for athletes. Physician Sportsmed. 13(3): 179, 1985.

Chapter 25

Andrews, J.R., and Harrelson, G.L.: Physical Rehabilitation of the Injured Athlete. Philadelphia, W.B. Saunders, 1991.

Gieck, J.H, and Saliba, E.N.: Application of modalities in overuse syndromes. Clin. Sports Med. 6: 127, 1987.

Hungerford, D.S., and Lennox, D.W.: Rehabilitation of the knee in disorders of the patellofemoral joint: Relevant biomechanics. Orthop. Clin. North Am. 14: 397, 1983.

Leadbetter, W.B., Buckwalter, J.A., and Gordon, S.L.(eds.): Sports-Induced Inflammation: Clinical and Basic Science Concepts. Park Ridge, IL, American Academy of Orthopaedic Surgeons, 1990.

McCue, F.C. III, and Mayer, V.: Rehabilitation of common athletic injuries of the hand and wrist. Clin. Sports Med. 8: 731, 1989.

Noyes, F.R., Butler, D.L., Paulos, L.E., and Grood, E.S.: Intra-articular cruciate reconstruction. I. Perspectives on graft strength, vascularization and immediate motion after replacement. Clin. Orthop. 172: 71, 1983.

Paulos, L.E.: Knee rehabilitation after anterior cruciate ligament reconstruction and repair. J. Orthop. Sports Phys. Ther. 13: 2, 1991.

Prentice, W.E.: Rehabilitation Techniques in Sports Medicine. St. Louis, Mosby College, 1990.

Reed, B., and Zarro, V.: Inflammation and repair and the use of thermal agents. In Thermal Agents in Rehabilitation. 2nd Ed. Edited by S.L. Michlovitz. Philadelphia, F.A. Davis, 1990.

Wright, C.S.: Tendon injuries in the hand and wrist. In Current Therapy in Sports Medicine, 2. Edited by J.S. Torg, R.P. Welsh, and R.J. Shephard. Philadelphia, B.C. Decker, 1990.

INDEX

Page numbers in *italics* indicate illustrations. Page numbers followed by a *t* indicate a table.

351